Oxford Case Histories in Infectious Diseases and Microbiology

Oxford Case Histories

Series Editors

Sarah Pendlebury and Peter Rothwell

Published:

Neurological Case Histories (Sarah T. Pendlebury, Philip Anslow, and Peter M. Rothwell)

Oxford Case Histories in Anaesthesia (Jon McCormack and Keith Kelly)

Oxford Case Histories in Cardiology (Rajkumar Rajendram, Javed Ehtisham, and ColinForfar)

Oxford Case Histories in Gastroenterology and Hepatology (Alissa J. Walsh, Otto C. Buchel, Jane Collier, and Simon P.L. Travis)

Oxford Case Histories in General Surgery (Judith Ritchie and K. Raj Prasad)

Oxford Case Histories in Geriatric Medicine (Sanja Thompson, Nicola Lovett, John Grimley Evans, and Sarah Pendlebury)

Oxford Case Histories in Lung Cancer (Himender K. Makker, Adam Ainley, Sanjay Popat, Julian Singer, Martin Hayward, and Antke Hagena)

Oxford Case Histories in Neurosurgery (Harutomo Hasegawa, Matthew Crocker, and Pawan Singh Minhas)

Oxford Case Histories in Oncology (Thankamma Ajithkumar, Adrian Harnett, and Tom Roques)

Oxford Case Histories in Respiratory Medicine (John Stradling, Andrew Stanton, Najib M. Rahman, Annabel H. Nickol, and Helen E. Davies)

Oxford Case Histories in Rheumatology (Joel David, Anne Miller, Anushka Soni, and Lyn Williamson)

Oxford Case Histories in Sleep Medicine (Himender K. Makker, Matthew Walker, Hugh Selsick, Bhik Kotecha, and Ama Johal)

Oxford Case Histories in TIA and Stroke (Sarah T. Pendlebury, Ursula G. Schulz, Aneil Malhotra, and Peter M. Rothwell)

Oxford Case Histories in Infectious Diseases and Microbiology

THIRD EDITION

Hilary Humphreys
William L. Irving
Bridget L. Atkins
Andrew F. Woodhouse

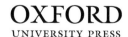

OXFORD
UNIVERSITY PRESS

OXFORD
UNIVERSITY PRESS

Great Clarendon Street, Oxford, OX2 6DP,
United Kingdom

Oxford University Press is a department of the University of Oxford.
It furthers the University's objective of excellence in research, scholarship,
and education by publishing worldwide. Oxford is a registered trade mark of
Oxford University Press in the UK and in certain other countries

© Oxford University Press 2020

The moral rights of the authors have been asserted

First Edition published by Churchill Livingston 1996
Second Edition published by Oxford University Press 2004
Third Edition published by Oxford University Press 2020

Published in the United States of America by Oxford University Press
198 Madison Avenue, New York, NY 10016, United States of America

British Library Cataloguing in Publication Data

Data available

Library of Congress Control Number: 2019948493

ISBN 978-0-19-884648-2

Printed and bound by
CPI Group (UK) Ltd, Croydon, CR0 4YY

Oxford University Press makes no representation, express or implied, that the
drug dosages in this book are correct. Readers must therefore always check
the product information and clinical procedures with the most up-to-date
published product information and data sheets provided by the manufacturers
and the most recent codes of conduct and safety regulations. The authors and
the publishers do not accept responsibility or legal liability for any errors in the
text or for the misuse or misapplication of material in this work. Except where
otherwise stated, drug dosages and recommendations are for the non-pregnant
adult who is not breast-feeding

Links to third party websites are provided by Oxford in good faith and
for information only. Oxford disclaims any responsibility for the materials
contained in any third party website referenced in this work.

A note from the series editors

Case histories have always had an important role in medical education, but most published material has been directed at undergraduates or residents. The Oxford Case Histories series aims to provide more complex case-based learning for clinicians in specialist training and consultants, and is now well-established in aiding preparation for entry- and exit-level specialty examinations and revalidation. Each case book follows the same format with approximately 45–50 cases, each comprising a brief clinical history and investigations, followed by questions on differential diagnosis and management, and detailed answers with discussion.

We are grateful to our colleagues in the various medical specialties for their enthusiasm and hard work in making the series possible.

Sarah Pendlebury and Peter Rothwell

From reviews of other books in the series:

Oxford Case Histories in Neurosurgery
'This book provides a great method for learning and preparing for neurosurgery examinations. The cases cover all relevant topics in neurosurgery, and the questions following the cases go to the core of the subject, highlighting the important points for students. The discussion section in particular is very informative, going over the differential diagnosis and citing the scientific basis for the answers. The strengths of the book are the simple and concise explanations and the discussions of related topics. This is useful not only for examinees, but also for practising neurosurgeons.'

Ramsis Farid Ghaly, MD, Doody's Notes

Oxford Case Histories in Cardiology

'Clearly the three authors have put a huge amount of time and effort into this book to make sure it is relevant, accurate and up to date.

   Overall, this book will be an excellent aid to those preparing for post-graduate exams in general medicine and cardiology, but will also be of relevance to senior medical students with more than a passing interest in cardiology.'

Cardiology News

Oxford Case Histories in Respiratory Medicine

'It is like having your favourite clinical teacher share his/her accumulated clinical nous in a way that makes the apparently ordinary case stimulating and full of subtlety ... I thoroughly enjoyed this book and recommend it to specialist registrars and consultants in respiratory medicine—go out and get a copy for your department.'

British Journal of Hospital Medicine

Oxford Case Histories in General Surgery

'The book has many strengths: it is supported by being part of a lineage of great pedigree, but it upholds the series' name with its own quality... This book has achieved everything it set out to do and I have enjoyed reading it.'

BMA reviewing panel, BMA Medical Book Awards

Preface

Infection continues to be important as a cause of admission to hospital and contributes to morbidity and mortality in the community. The re-emergence of diseases, previously thought to be quiescent, such as Ebola, and new challenges, for example, carbapenemase-producing Enterobacteriaceae (Enterobacterales), mean that there is almost constant change and a need to adapt and amend current approaches to diagnosis, management, and prevention.

Case histories are a useful learning medium as they reflect, to some degree, real life; patients present with a constellation of symptoms and signs which suggest infection and warrant further investigation and management. Our choice of cases is meant to reflect important pathogens and disease syndromes as well as those that are either common or critical in terms of an adverse outcome. However, not every particular pathogen or infection syndrome can be covered in this format. Rather, the cases we have included reflect the priorities of the authors as to what the trainee should be familiar with and those areas discussed in each case are currently of interest or reflect where there is controversy. Each case in addition is followed by further reading with approximately five sources listed where the reader may find additional information germane to that covered in the text.

While this set of case histories is primarily designed for trainees in clinical microbiology, clinical virology and infectious diseases, it will also be of interest to those working in critical care medicine, public health, and paediatrics.

The authors would like to thank their colleagues for helpful advice, for reading drafts, providing illustrations, and for their support and inspiration. We have acknowledged those in person who have contributed. We would also like to thank Caroline Smith from Oxford University Press for her advice, support, and patience during the drafting of the case series.

We hope you find the book useful, the case histories informative, and that you continue to be as fascinated by the myriad range of infections and microbes that are to be encountered, as we ourselves continue to be.

Hilary Humphreys, William L. Irving, Bridget L. Atkins,
and Andrew F. Woodhouse

Contents

Abbreviations

¹⁸F-FDG-PET-CT	¹⁸F-fluorodeoxyglucose-Positron Emission Tomography-Computerized Tomography		CDI	*Clostridioides* (*Clostridium*) *difficile* infection
			CF	cystic fibrosis
			CL	cutaneous leishmaniasis
AGNB	aerobic Gram-negative bacilli		CMV	cytomegalovirus
			CNS	central nervous system
AIDS	acquired immunodeficiency syndrome		CoNS	coagulase-negative staphylococci
			COPD	chronic obstructive pulmonary disease
ALT	Alanine transaminase		CPE	Carbapenemase Producing Enterobacteriacae (Enterobacterales)
AOSD	adult-onset Stills disease			
APC	antigen presenting cells			
APRI	aspartate aminotransferase to platelet ratio index		CRB-65	Confusion, Respiratory rate, Blood pressure, age 65 or over
			CRE	Carbapenem-resistant Enterobacterales
ART	antiretroviral therapy			
ASOT	anti-streptolysin O titre		CRP	C-reactive protein
AS	acute schistosomiasis		CSF	cerebrospinal fluid
AST	aspartate transaminase		CT	computerized tomography
AST	American Society of Transplantation		CURB-65	Confusion, Urea, Respiratory rate, Blood pressure, age 65 or over
BAL	broncho-alveolar lavage			
BBV	blood-borne virus		CXR	chest X-ray
BCNIE	blood culture-negative infective endocarditis		DAAs	direct-acting antiviral agents
			DAIR	debridement, antibiotics, and implant retention
bd	twice daily			
bd po	twice daily by mouth		DFI	diabetic foot infection
BKVAN	BK virus-associated nephropathy		DNA	deoxyribonucleic acid
			DST	drug susceptibility testing
BMI	body mass index		DTP	differential time to positivity
BSI	bloodstream infection		EAEC	enteroaggregative *E. coli*
CA-MRSA	community-acquired methicillin-resistant *S. aureus*		EBV	Epstein–Barr virus
			ECDC	European Centre for Disease Control
CAP	community-acquired pneumonia		ECG	electrocardiogram
			ED	Emergency Department
CAPD	continuous ambulatory peritoneal dialysis		EIA	enzyme immuno-assay

ELF	enhanced liver fibrosis		IFN	interferon
ELISA	enzyme-linked immunosorbent assay		Ig	immunoglobulin
			IHA	indirect haemagglutination assay
EOT	end of treatment		IID	infectious intestinal disease
EPP	exposure-prone procedure		IPD	invasive pneumococcal disease
EPS	extracellular polymeric substances		IU	international units
			IV	intravenous
ESBL	extended-spectrum β-lactamases		IVIG	intravenous immunoglobulin
ETEC	enterotoxigenic *E. coli*		IVS	identified validated sample
EVD	Ebola virus disease		JCV	JC virus
EVD	extra-ventricular drain		KDIGO	Kidney Disease: Improving Global Outcomes
FBC	full blood count		LFT	liver function test
FFP	filtering facepiece (mask)		LP	lumbar puncture
FMT	faecal microbiota transplantation		LPAI	low pathogenicity avian influenza
GAS	Group A streptococci		MAC	*Mycobacterium avium* complex
GCS	Glasgow Coma Scale			
GP	General Practitioner		MALDI-TOF	matrix-assisted laser desorption/ionization time-of-flight mass spectrometry
HACEK	*Haemophilus* spp., *Aggregatibacter actinomycetemcomitans.*, *Cardiobacterium hominis*, *Eikenella corrodens*, and *Kingella kingae*		MDR-TB	multi-drug-resistant tuberculosis
			MDT	multidisciplinary team
HBV	Hepatitis B virus		MERS-CoV	Middle Eastern Respiratory Syndrome corona virus
HCV	Hepatitis C virus			
HDU	high dependency unit		MHC	major histocompatibility complex
HEV	Hepatitis E virus			
HIV	human immunodeficiency virus		MIC	minimum inhibitory concentration
HHV	human herpes virus			
HLH	haemophagocytic lymphohistiocytosis		ML	mucosal leishmaniasis
			MLST	multilocus sequence typing
HPS	Hantavirus pulmonary syndrome		MMR	measles, mumps, rubella
			MRI	magnetic resonance imaging
HSCT	haematopoietic stem cell transplant		MRSA	methicillin-resistant *Staphylococcus aureus*
HSV	herpes simplex virus			
IA	immuno-assay		MS	multiple sclerosis
ICP	intracranial pressure		MSIS	Musculoskeletal Infection Society
ICU	intensive care unit			
IDSA	Infectious Diseases Society of America		MSSA	methicillin-susceptible *Staphylococcus aureus*
IE	infective endocarditis		NAFLD	non-alcoholic fatty liver disease

NBTE	non-bacterial thrombotic endocarditis		RCOG	Royal College of Obstetricians and Gynaecologists
NDM	New Delhi metallo-β-lactamase		RdRp	RNA-dependent RNA polymerase
NICE	National Institute for Health and Care Excellence		RDT	rapid diagnostic tests
NICU	neurosurgical intensive care unit		RNA	ribonucleic acid
			ROI	reduction of immunosuppression
NHS	National Health Service			
NMN	Novy–McNeal–Nicolle (media)		RT-PCR	reverse transcriptase PCR
od	once daily		SAB	*S. aureus* bloodstream (infection)
OH	Occupational Health			
OPAT	Out-patient Parenteral Antibiotic Therapy		SARS	Severe Acute Respiratory Syndrome
PAS	*p*-aminosalicylic acid		SEM	skin, eye, and mouth
PAS	periodic acid-Schiff		SLE	systemic lupus erythematosis
PCR	polymerase chain reaction		SOT	solid organ transplant
PEG-IFN	pegylated IFN		SPE	streptococcal pyrogenic exotoxins
PET	Positron Emission Tomography			
PHE	Public Health England		SSPE	sub-acute sclerosing panencephalitis
PI	protease inhibitor		SVR	sustained virologic response
PICC	peripherally inserted central catheter		TB	tuberculosis
			TC	T cells
PML	progressive multifocal leukoencephalopathy		TCR	T cell receptor
			TD	traveller's diarrhoea
PPE	personal protective equipment		TSS	toxic shock syndrome
PPJI	peri-prosthetic joint infection		USS	ultrasonography scan
PPV	pneumococcal polysaccharide vaccine		VHF	viral haemorrhagic fever
			VPS	ventriculo-peritoneal shunt
PTLD	post-transplant lymphoproliferative disease		VZV	varicella-zoster virus
PUO	pyrexia of unknown origin		VZIG	varicella-zoster immune globulin
PVL	Panton–Valentine leukocidin			
RAPD	Random Amplification of Polymorphic DNA		WCC	white blood cell count
			WGS	whole genome sequencing
RAS	resistance associated substitution		WHO	World Health Organization
			XDR-TB	extensively drug-resistant tuberculosis
RBV	ribavirin			

Authors

Hilary Humphreys, Professor of Clinical Microbiology and Consultant in Microbiology, RCSI Education and Research Centre, Beaumont Hospital, Dublin, Ireland

William L. Irving, Professor and Honorary Consultant in Virology, University of Nottingham and Nottingham University Hospitals NHS Trust, UK

Bridget L. Atkins, Consultant in Microbiology and Infectious Diseases, Oxford University Hospitals NHS Foundation Trust and Training Programme Director, Health Education England (Thames Valley), UK

Andrew F. Woodhouse, Consultant in Infectious Diseases, University Hospitals Birmingham NHS Foundation Trust and Training Programme Director, Health Education England (West Midlands), UK

Contributors

Bridget L. Atkins, Consultant in Microbiology and Infectious Diseases, Oxford University Hospitals NHS Foundation Trust and Training Programme Director, Health Education England (Thames Valley), UK
Cases: 12, 29, 42, and 43

Lucinda Barrett, Consultant in Microbiology, Oxford University Hospitals NHS Foundation Trust, UK
Cases: 29 and 43

Hilary Humphreys, Professor of Clinical Microbiology and Consultant in Microbiology, RCSI Education and Research Centre, Beaumont Hospital, Dublin, Ireland
Cases: 1, 4, 5, 7, 8, 13, 14, 15, 17, 23, 26, 27, 28, 34, 41, and 47

William L. Irving, Professor and Honorary Consultant in Virology, University of Nottingham and Nottingham University Hospitals NHS Trust, UK
Cases: 20, 21, and 44

Katie Jeffery, Consultant in Microbiology, Oxford University Hospitals NHS Foundation Trust, UK
Case: 39

Nicola Jones, Consultant in Infectious Diseases and General Medicine, Oxford University Hospitals NHS Foundation Trust, UK
Case: 9

Seilesh Kadambari, Clinical Lecturer, Department of Paediatrics, University of Oxford, UK
Case: 40

Maheshi Ramasamy, Consultant in Infectious Diseases and General Medicine, Oxford University Hospitals NHS Foundation Trust, UK
Cases: 2, 6, 22, and 32

T H Nicholas Wong, Consultant in Microbiology and Infectious Diseases, Buckinghamshire Healthcare NHS Trust, UK
Cases: 19, 24, and 33

Andrew F. Woodhouse, Consultant in Infectious Diseases, University Hospitals Birmingham NHS Foundation Trust and Training Programme Director, Health Education England (West Midlands), UK
Cases: 3, 10, 11, 16, 18, 25, 30, 35, 36, 37, 45, and 46

Table of normal ranges

Text	Value	Unit
Haemoglobin (Hb)	12–16 (women), 13–17 (men)	g/dl
WCC	4–11	10^9/l
Neutrophils	2–7	10^9/l
Lymphocytes	1–4	10^9/l
Platelets	150–400	10^9/l
ESR	<20 (women), <14 (men)	mm/h
aPTT	26–36	sec
PT	13–16	sec
Vit B12	180–900	ng/l
Folate	4–24	µg/l
Sodium (Na)	135–145	mmol/l
Potassium (K)	3.5–5.0	mmol/l
Urea (U)	2.5–6.7	mmol/l
Creatinine (Cr)	70–150	µmol/l
Glucose	3.0–5.5 (fasting)	mmol/l
C-reactive Protein (CRP)	<8	mg/l
Bilirubin	3–17	µmol/l
ALT	10–45	iU/l
AST	15–42	iU/l
Alkaline phosphatase (Alk P)	95–320	iU/l
Albumin	35–50	g/l
γ-GT	15–40	iU/l
Creatine Kinase (CK)	24–195	iU/l
IgG	6.0–13.0	g/l
IgA	0.8–3.0	g/l
IgM	0.4–2.5	g/l
CD4	500–1,500	cells/mm^3
Ferritin	15–200	µg/l

Text	Value	Unit
Blood gases		
PH	7.35–7.45	
Partial pressure of oxygen (PaO₂)	>10.6	KPa
Partial pressure of carbon dioxide (PaCO₂)	4.7–.60	KPa
Bicarbonate	24–30	mmol/L
Cerebrospinal fluid		
WBC	<5	cells per μl
Protein	150–400	mg/l
Glucose	at least 60% of serum glucose	mmol/l
Opening pressure	7–18	cm H₂O

Adapted with permission from Pendlebury S. T. et al. (2012). *Oxford Case Histories in TIA and Stroke*. Oxford, UK: Oxford University Press.

Section 1

Skin and soft tissue infections

Case 1

Hilary Humphreys

Case history

A 67-year-old female presents to the Emergency Department (ED) with a spreading area of erythema on the right thigh and related pain. She has a background history of a total hip replacement five years earlier and has stable ischaemic heart disease. On examination, she has a body mass index (BMI) of 40.6, her blood pressure and respiratory rate are normal, but she has a temperature of 39.5 °C. Her physical examination is unremarkable apart from a well-demarcated area of erythema on the right thigh that is hot to touch (Fig. 1.1). There are no blisters or any evidence of necrosis/gangrene.

Questions

1.1 Is this likely to be cellulitis, erysipelas, or necrotizing fasciitis?

1.2 What are the most likely causes?

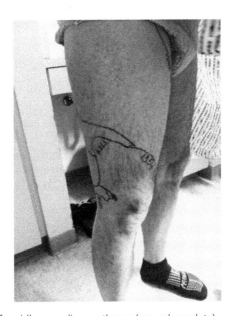

Figure 1.1 Area of rapidly spreading erythema (see colour plate).

Answers

1.1 Is this likely to be cellulitis, erysipelas, or necrotizing fasciitis?

Cellulitis involves infection of the dermis and subcutaneous tissues whereas erysipelas is more superficial and involves the dermal structures only. There is often clear demarcation between affected and non-affected skin and raised borders, with erysipelas. In contrast, necrotizing fasciitis involves skin and deeper layers, especially fascia, and may be characterized by blisters and necrotic tissue. It is also associated with severe pain and is a surgical emergency. Therefore, the case described here is most likely to be cellulitis.

1.2 What are the most likely causes?

Cellulitis associated with pus or abscesses is most likely to be due to *Staphylococcus aureus* including community-acquired methicillin-resistant *S. aureus* (CA-MRSA). However, in the absence of pus, β-haemolytic streptococci such as group A streptococci (GAS) (or *Streptococcus pyogenes*) are the most likely cause. Occasionally cellulitis may be polymicrobial and involve Gram-negative bacilli and anaerobes, but not typically.

Case history continued

On the basis of the clinical examination a diagnosis of cellulitis is made. It transpires that she has been on co-amoxiclav, which was started by her General Practitioner (GP) five days earlier when she initially presented but the cellulitis has spread despite the antibiotic. She also describes having a similar episode two years ago.

She is started on high-dose intravenous flucloxacillin and the co-amoxiclav is discontinued. Blood cultures are sterile and she remains clinically stable. The patient slowly responds to treatment and is discharged home on oral antibiotics. However, within the next 10 days, two further patients present on the same ward develop cellulitis, and one has a positive blood culture for GAS. An outbreak team is convened to investigate the possibility of hospital-acquired acquisition of GAS.

Questions

1.3 What microbiological investigations are indicated in cellulitis?

1.4 Should the original patient also receive benzylpenicillin?

1.5 For how long should this patient be treated?

1.6 Should healthcare workers be screened for GAS during an outbreak investigation?

1.7 When can a healthcare worker positive for GAS go back to work?

1.8 Should the initial patient described here receive prophylactic antibiotics?

Answers

1.3 What microbiological investigations are indicated in cellulitis?

Blood cultures, needle aspirates of fluid, and skin biopsies may reveal the diagnosis. However, the yield from blood cultures is usually less than 10% and even an aspirate from the advancing edge of the cellulitis may not be positive. Skin biopsies, rarely done in practice, may provide a microbiological diagnosis in up to a quarter of cases. In addition, recent/current antibiotics as in the case described will reduce the yield from cultures. An anti-streptolysin O titre (ASOT) may retrospectively support a diagnosis of GAS infection. Molecular diagnostic approaches such as polymerase chain reaction (PCR) amplification of the 16S rDNA gene followed by cloning and sequencing (Case 35) may be helpful but this is not yet validated in routine practice. It is usual to type the isolate if it is GAS for epidemiological purposes. Some strains are more virulent than others. If the responsible bacterium is *S. aureus*, the presence of Panton–Valentine leukocidin (PVL) is sometimes investigated for as it may be associated with severe invasive disease.

1.4 Should the original patient also receive benzylpenicillin?

No. There is no convincing evidence to support the addition of benzylpenicillin, to cover GAS in addition to high-dose flucloxacillin. If GAS is subsequently confirmed as the cause, flucloxacillin can be changed to benzylpenicillin. If MRSA is initially suspected either because of a poor response to initial treatment or because of the presence of risk factors for community-acquired methicillin-resistant *S. aureus* (CA-MRSA)—that is, close contact and cuts with compromised skin integrity—then an antibiotic with MRSA activity such as vancomycin/teicoplanin should be started. In the absence of a microbiology diagnosis, definitive treatment is challenging. Agents used to cover MRSA and streptococci also include linezolid, daptomycin, and clindamycin (Table 1.1). In particular, clindamycin and linezolid suppress toxin production and are often given in combination with flucloxacillin if severe or if necrotizing fasciitis is suspected.

1.5 For How long should this patient be treated?

The optimal duration of antibiotics for cellulitis is unknown. Most agree that at least 5–10 days are required but sometimes antibiotics may be continued for 2–3 weeks. However, depending on the antibiotic susceptibility of the isolate, an intravenous (IV) to oral switch may occur if the patient is stable, if there is an oral option, and the patient does not need IV treatment for other reasons. A need for intravenous treatment in a stable patient may be met by an out-patient antibiotic therapy (OPAT) service but this requires close monitoring and compliance with antimicrobial

Table 1.1 Alternative/newer antibiotic options available to treat streptococcal/ staphylococcal cellulitis

Agents	Advantages	Disadvantages	Comments
Doxycline	Can be administered orally after discharge	MRSA isolates may be resistant	Contra-indicated during pregnancy
Trimethoprim-sulfamethoxazole	Used in North America to treat MRSA	Side-effect profile of sulphonamides	Careful choice of dosing compared to that for pneumocystis pneumonia
Linezolid	Oral and IV administration. Good tissue penetration and suppresses toxin production	Myelosuppression, optic neuritis, and drug interactions	Resistance may emerge and concern about long-term use
Daptomycin	Bactericidal and once-daily administration	Myopathy and rhabdomyolysis	Be aware of cross-resistance with vancomycin
Dalbavancin	Long half-life with a once-weekly two-dose regimen	More haemorrhagic effects than comparator drugs in trials	Still being evaluated outside of initial trials. May be used as part of OPAT regimens or in the ED
Ceftaroline fosamil	Broad-spectrum cephalosporin with activity against MRSA	Risk of *Clostridium difficile* as with other cephalosporins	Not widely available and or used

OPAT, out-patient antibiotic therapy; ED, Emergency Department.

stewardship policies. Adjuvant treatment for cellulitis caused by GAS that have been considered include corticosteroids and intravenous immunoglobulin. However, the evidence for these is poor.

1.6 Should healthcare workers be screened for GAS during an outbreak investigation?

There is no definite answer to this question. All cases of invasive GAS should be notified to public health as soon possible. Less than 5% of the adult population carry GAS, but asymptomatic healthcare workers may transmit this bacterium particularly if they have skin lesions. A decision to screen healthcare workers must involve occupational health who are best positioned to carry out the screening and explain the consequences to any positive staff members.

1.7 When can a healthcare worker positive for GAS go back to work?

Usually a staff member can go back to work when they have had at least 24 hours of appropriate treatment, for example penicillin V or clindamycin.

1.8 Should the initial patient described here receive prophylactic antibiotics?

Probably. Up to 30% of patients with cellulitis may develop a recurrence. Systematic reviews suggest that antibiotic prophylaxis significantly reduces the number of patients with recurrent cellulitis but the duration of prophylaxis is variable. Usually, either an oral penicillin or a macrolide is used. This patient has had two episodes of cellulitis and therefore may be a candidate for prophylaxis.

Further reading

Fogo A, Kemp N, Morris-Jones R. PVL positive *Staphylococcus aureus* skin infections. *Br Med J* 2011; **343**: d5343 doi:10.1136/bmj.d5343.

Gilchrist M, Seaton RA. Outpatient parenteral antimicrobial therapy and antimicrobial stewardship: challenges and checklists. *J Antimicrob Chemother* 2015; **70**: 965–70.

Oh CC, Ko HCH, Lee HY, Safdar N, Maki DG, et al. Antibiotic prophylaxis for preventing recurrent cellulitis: a systematic review and meta-analysis. *J Infect* 2014; **69**: 26–34.

Raff AB, Kroshinsky D. Cellulitis a review. *J Am Med Ass* 2016; **316**: 325–337.

Steer JA, Lamagni T, Healy B, Morgan M, Dryden M, et al. Guidelines for prevention and control of group A streptococcal infection in acute healthcare and maternity settings in the UK. *J Infect* 2012; **64**: 1–18.

Case 2

Maheshi Ramasamy

Case history

A previously well 55-year-old woman is brought in to the Emergency Department (ED) by ambulance, having collapsed at home. On arrival she is drowsy, vomiting, and hypotensive with a blood pressure of 75/50 and a temperature of 39.8 °C. Key findings on examination are: a 2 cm × 1 cm furuncle on her foot with some surrounding erythema which was sustained after a recent gardening accident; a macular erythematous rash across her abdomen, neck, and back; and conjunctival injection. She has been anuric for the past 12 hours. A presumptive diagnosis of toxic shock syndrome (TSS) is made. Initial laboratory investigations reveal a metabolic acidosis, acute renal failure, and a transaminitis. The patient is transferred to intensive care for further management.

Questions

2.1 What is the pathogenesis of TSS?

2.2 How is TSS diagnosed?

2.3 What is the immediate management of this patient?

2.4 What is the role of intravenous immunoglobulin (IVIG) in the treatment of TSS?

Answers

2.1 What is the pathogenesis of TSS?

TSS is a clinical syndrome characterized by shock and multi-organ failure and is mediated by bacterial toxins which act as immunological superantigens (Fig. 2.1). Superantigens stimulate large pools of T cells simultaneously, resulting in high

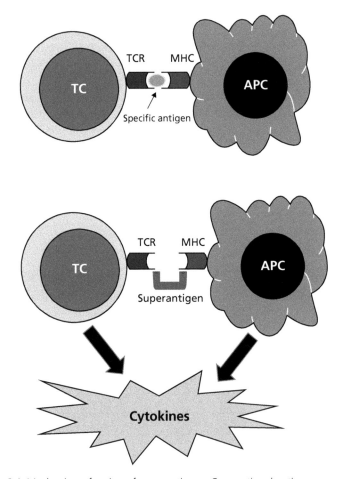

Figure 2.1 Mechanism of action of superantigens. Conventional antigens are displayed on major histocompatibility complex (MHC) molecules by antigen presenting cells (APC) to T cells (TC). TC recognize the antigen-MHC complex via specific T cell receptors (TCR). This results in activation of relatively few subsets of antigen specific TC. Superantigens, however, cross-link MHC and the TCR directly, irrespective of TC specificity. This results in the activation of up to 30% of all circulating TC and hence massive inflammatory cytokine release, resulting in capillary leak and tissue damage.

circulating levels of inflammatory cytokines such as IL-1, IL-2, and TNFα. The former causes fever, the latter two increase capillary permeability, which in turn leads to profound hypotension, tissue hypoperfusion, and organ failure.

TSS was first described in relation to *Staphylococcus aureus* infection. The *S. aureus* exotoxin toxic shock syndrome toxin 1 (TSST-1) is implicated in most cases. Approximately half of staphylococcal TSS cases are related to menstruation, with the use of high-absorbency tampons being a risk factor for disease. Non-menstrual staphylococcal TSS cases are associated with surgical or obstetric wound infections, skin lesions, or recent respiratory virus infections. Host factors play an important role in the pathogenesis of TSS—patients with TSS fail to mount an anti-body response to TSST-1, while measurable titres are found in women colonized with TSST-1 producing strains of *S. aureus*. Thus, an absence of a protective anti-body response to TSST-1 may correlate with disease.

Group A streptococci (*Streptococcus pyogenes* or GAS) can also cause TSS. The streptococcal pyrogenic exotoxins (SPE) types A, B, and C are analogous to TSST-1 and act as superantigens, initiating cytokine production. Streptococcal TSS is most commonly associated with invasive infections such as necrotizing fasciitis, blood-stream infection (BSI), or pneumonia, rather than the more common manifestations of streptococcal disease such as pharyngitis or skin/soft tissue infection.

TSS can also be caused by other streptococcal species possessing SPE or occasion-ally by *Clostridium* spp.

2.2 How is TSS diagnosed?

Clinical manifestations of TSS include fever, hypotension, and skin manifestations (Tables 2.1 and 2.2). Laboratory tests reflect shock and end organ damage. The iso-lation of *S. aureus* is not required for the diagnosis of staphylococcal TSS, although it may be recovered from wound or mucosal sites in up to 80% of patients. These isolates may be tested for toxin production in reference laboratories. In addition, acute and convalescent serum can be screened for antibody to TSST-1. Isolation of GAS from a sterile site is a prerequisite for the diagnosis of streptococcal TSS.

Although many of the clinical manifestations of staphylococcal and streptococcal TSS are similar, there are a few key differences. In streptococcal TSS, the mortality is higher (30% versus 3% with *S. aureus*), BSI and tissue necrosis are more common, and generalized erythema is less common.

2.3 What is the immediate management of this patient?

The treatment of TSS involves management of septic shock and its complications, antibiotic therapy, and source control.

Patients may require aggressive fluid resuscitation and vasopressors and for this reason are best managed in the critical care setting.

Infective foci—for example, retained tampons, surgical dressings—should be sought and removed. Prompt surgical exploration and debridement of soft tissue

Table 2.1 Clinical diagnosis of staphylococcal toxic shock syndrome

Diagnosis of staphylococcal toxic shock syndrome	
Clinical criteria (all five must be present unless patient dies before desquamation occurs)	1. **Fever** ≥ 38.9 °C
	2. **Rash** diffuse, macular
	3. **Desquamation** 1–2 weeks after onset of rash
	4. **Hypotension** (SBP ≤ 90 mmHg)
	5. **Multi-system involvement** **To include three or more of:** ♦ Renal dysfunction ♦ Coagulopathy ♦ Liver dysfunction ♦ Gastrointestinal symptoms (e.g. vomiting/diarrhoea) ♦ Mucous membrane involvement (e.g. oropharyngeal/conjunctival hyperaemia) ♦ Central nervous system dysfunction (e.g. disorientation, altered consciousness) ♦ Muscular (e.g. myalgia or raised creatinine kinase)
Laboratory criteria	Negative blood or cerebrospinal fluid cultures for another pathogen (may be positive for *S. aureus*, but not essential) **AND** Negative serology for Rocky Mountain Spotted Fever (in endemic areas), leptospirosis, measles

Adapted from Centers for Disease Control and Prevention (CDC). *Toxic Shock Syndrome (other than streptococcal) (TSS) 2011 Case Definition*. Atlanta, GA: CDC. http://wwwn.cdc.gov/nndss/conditions/toxic-shock-syndrome-other-than-streptococcal/case-definition/2011/.

Table 2.2 Clinical diagnosis of streptococcal toxic shock syndrome

Diagnosis of streptococcal toxic shock syndrome	
Laboratory criteria	Isolation of GAS from a normally sterile site (e.g. blood, cerebrospinal fluid, tissue biopsy)
Clinical severity criteria	Hypotension (SBP ≤ 90 mmHg) **AND 2 OR MORE OF** ♦ Renal dysfunction ♦ Coagulopathy ♦ Liver dysfunction ♦ Acute respiratory distress syndrome ♦ Erythematous rash (may desquamate) ♦ Soft tissue necrosis (e.g. necrotizing fasciitis or myositis)

Source: data from Breiman, RF et al. (1993). Defining the group A streptococcal toxic shock syndrome. *JAMA* 269(3): 390–1. DOI:10.1001/jama.1993.03500030088038.

infection may be required, particularly if underlying tissue necrosis is suspected. This patient's foot lesion was surgically debrided and intraoperative samples subsequently grew a methicillin-susceptible *Staphylococcus aureus*.

Empiric antibiotic therapy in general should include a cell wall agent, such as an appropriate β-lactam. This should be initially in combination with intravenous clindamycin, which inhibits protein synthesis. *In vitro* experiments demonstrate that by inhibiting protein synthesis, clindamycin inhibits toxin production and the production of other virulence factors. Although no randomized trials exist for antibiotic regimens in the treatment of TSS, these experimental data and further observational studies support the use of combination therapy with clindamycin.

2.4 What is the role of intravenous immunoglobulin (IVIG) in the treatment of TSS?

The largest body of evidence for the use of IVIG is in the setting of streptococcal TSS. IVIG is postulated to neutralize SPE and other streptococcal virulence factors as well as having direct immunomodulatory effects. Observational studies suggest that adjunctive IVIG therapy may improve survival in streptococcal TSS and for this reason it may be administered in patients with refractory shock. There are few published studies on the use of IVIG in staphylococcal TSS, although *in vitro* studies suggest higher doses may be required than for streptococcal TSS.

Further reading

Centers for Disease Control. Toxic Shock Syndrome (other than streptococcal) (TSS) 2011 Case Definition [Internet]. Atlanta, GA: CDC. Available at: http://wwwn.cdc.gov/nndss/conditions/toxic-shock-syndrome-other-than-streptococcal/case-definition/2011/ accessed 21 July 2019.

Linnér A, Darenberg J, Sjölin J, Henriques-Normark B, Norrby-Teglund A. Clindamycin Affects Group A Streptococcus Virulence Factors and Improves Clinical Outcome. *J Infect Dis* 2016; **0**. doi: jiw229v2–jiw229.

Linnér A, Darenberg J, Sjölin J, Henriques-Normark B, Norrby-Teglund A. Clinical efficacy of polyspecific intravenous immunoglobulin therapy in patients with streptococcal toxic shock syndrome: A comparative observational study. *Clin Infect Dis* 2014; **59**: 851–7.

Stevens D. The toxic shock syndromes. *Infect Dis Clin North Am* 1996; **10**: 727.

The Working Group on Severe Streptococcal Infections. Defining the group A streptococcal toxic shock syndrome. Rationale and consensus definition. *JAMA* 1993; **269**: 390.

Case 3

Andrew Woodhouse

Case history

A 35-year-old man presents with fever and a rash (Fig. 3.1) consisting of vesicles with surrounding erythema involving predominantly his face and trunk which began two days previously. He has no underlying medical problems but smokes 20 cigarettes per day. Over the last 24 hours new vesicles have been appearing and he has become more unwell and is complaining of cough, chest tightness, and breathlessness on minor exertion. Sixteen days previously he had attended his nephew's third birthday party and he has been told that one of the children attending developed chicken pox the day after the event.

His respiratory rate is 26 per minute and oxygen saturation on room air is 88%. An arterial blood gas shows a pO_2 of 8.5 kPa on air. A chest X-ray (CXR) (Fig. 3.2) is obtained.

Questions

3.1 What is the likely diagnosis?

3.2 How can the diagnosis be confirmed and what further investigations are indicated at this point?

3.3 What is the likely cause of the CXR appearance?

3.4 How should he be managed and what antimicrobial treatment, if any, is indicated?

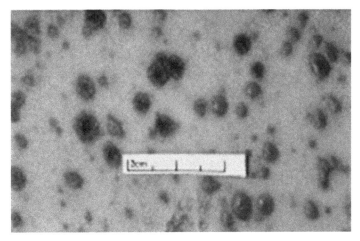

Figure 3.1 Vesicular rash (see colour plate).

Reproduced courtesy of David Warrell, Emeritus Professor of Tropical Medicine, Nuffield Department of Clinical Medicine, Oxford, UK.

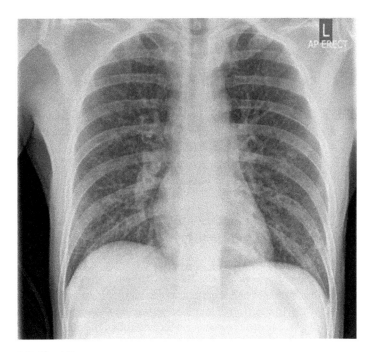

Figure 3.2 Chest X-ray.

Reproduced courtesy of University Hospitals Birmingham NHS Foundation Trust, UK.

3.1 What is the likely diagnosis?

Varicella (chicken pox) is the most likely diagnosis based on the appearance of the rash (Fig. 3.1) and exposure history. Varicella is highly transmissible to susceptible hosts and the infectivity period begins 48 hours before the appearance of the rash and continues until lesions have fully crusted. The incubation period is variable but on average is typically 2 weeks from exposure with a range of between 10 and 21 days.

3.2 How can the diagnosis be confirmed and what further investigations are indicated at this point?

Most often the diagnosis is made clinically but laboratory confirmation is by detection of varicella-zoster virus (VZV) by PCR of fluid or tissue from a vesicle. The majority of patients with uncomplicated varicella are managed in the community and do not require any investigations. In this case the patient's respiratory symptoms suggest possible varicella pneumonia as a complication and he requires further work-up. A CXR and an assessment of his respiratory function are required. Routine blood tests such as full blood count (FBC), renal, and liver function are reasonable. Careful examination of his skin to exclude bacterial infection and a neurological examination should be documented.

3.3 What is the likely cause of the CXR appearance?

The CXR is consistent with varicella pneumonia and shows patchy bilateral reticulonodular infiltrates. This complication of varicella is more common in adults than children with an incidence of about 1 in 400 cases. Smoking, immunosuppression, pregnancy, and male gender have been identified as risk factors for developing varicella pneumonia. It is associated with significant mortality (10–25%) which can rise to close to 50% in patients unwell enough to require mechanical ventilation.

3.4 How should he be managed and what antimicrobial treatment, if any, is indicated?

He has complicated varicella infection and requires admission to hospital for close monitoring, oxygen therapy, supportive care, and antiviral treatment. He is infectious as he has vesicles which have not yet crusted and should be nursed in respiratory isolation. Aciclovir, valaciclovir, and famciclovir are the antivirals commonly used to treat varicella. Due to the poor oral bioavailability of aciclovir, the newer agents valaciclovir and famciclovir are used in oral treatment as they achieve the required drug levels with more reliability.

While uncomplicated varicella is generally self-limiting in children and adults, aciclovir treatment does shorten the duration of symptoms and time to recovery in adults if started early, that is, within 24 hours of the appearance of rash. For this reason, early treatment is generally recommended although it remains unclear, due to a paucity of data, whether the frequency of complications is reduced by treatment.

Treatment is indicated in this case due to the presence of pneumonia. In complicated and severe varicella, antiviral treatment is recommended irrespective of the time of presentation relative to the initial appearance of rash. In complicated disease and in immunocompromised hosts intravenous aciclovir is preferred initially at a dose of 10 mg/kg 8 hourly. Treatment is usually continued for at least 7 days although switching to a well-absorbed oral agent may be an option when improvement is noted.

Case history continued

The patient is admitted and managed initially in a high dependency unit (HDU) due to increasing oxygen requirements. PCR confirms VZV and over the next 48 hours he begins to improve with fever abating and stable oxygen requirements. On the fourth day of admission he becomes febrile again and has a rigor. He becomes hypotensive and has a persistent tachycardia. No new vesicles have developed since starting treatment and most of the existing lesions are crusted but a patch of erythema is noted over his trunk which has enlarged over the course of the day and this is diagnosed as cellulitis.

The patient is concerned because a friend of his who visited him for the day 24 hours prior to him developing the rash is 18 weeks pregnant. The friend does not know whether she has had chickenpox in the past and she has never been vaccinated.

Questions

3.5 What is the likely organism causing the cellulitis?

3.6 What advice should be offered to his pregnant friend about the risk?

3.7 Would any investigation be appropriate for her?

Answers

3.5 What is the likely organism causing the cellulitis?

Varicella is associated with an increased incidence of skin and soft tissue infection caused by Group A streptococci (*S. pyogenes*). A range of manifestations is observed from cellulitis to more invasive disease including necrotizing fasciitis, BSI, and streptococcal toxic shock syndrome (Case 2). Management of sepsis and appropriate antibiotics are required.

3.6 What advice should be offered to his pregnant friend about the risk?

The friend has had a significant face-to-face contact during the infectious period and therefore is at risk of having acquired infection if she in not immune. The risk analysis is influenced by her pregnancy, both in terms of a predisposition to more severe disease if she has been infected and the risk to the foetus. Congenital varicella syndrome is a potential risk if infection develops in the mother during early pregnancy.

3.7 Would any investigation be appropriate for her?

Yes. Varicella serology should be obtained. If she is seropositive she is considered immune and no further action is required. If she is seronegative and still within 10 days of exposure she might be offered passive immunization with varicella-zoster immune globulin (VZIG). At times of VZIG shortage in the United Kingdom, this is reserved for women less than 20 weeks pregnant. Those more than 20 weeks should be offered acyclovir 7–14 days after contact. This strategy reduces the risk of developing infection and also decreases the severity of infection in those who develop disease in spite of passive immunization. VZIG also reduces the likelihood of congenital varicella if the woman develops chickenpox despite prophylaxis.

Further reading

Cohen J, Breuer J. Chickenpox: treatment. *Br Med J Clin Evid* 2015; Jun 15: pii:0912.

Gershon AA, Breuer J, Cohen JI, Cohrs RJ, Gershon MD, et al. Varicella zoster virus infection. *Nat Rev Dis Primers* 2015; **60**: 1068–74. https://www.gov.uk/government/collections/chickenpox-public-health-management-and-guidance accessed 21 July 2019.

Mirouse A, Vignon P, Piron P, Robert R, Papazian L, et al. Severe varicella-zoster virus pneumonia: a multi-center cohort study. *Crit Care* 2017; **21**: 137. doi: 10.1186/s 13054-017-1731-0.

Public Health England. Chickenpox: public health management and guidance. The diagnosis, management and epidemiology of chickenpox (varicella). 2014. https://www.gov.uk/government/collections/chickenpox-public-health-management-and-guidance accessed 21 July 2019.

Tunbridge AJ, Breuer J, Jeffery KJM. Chicken pox in adults—clinical management. *J Infection* 2008; **57**: 95–102.

Case 4

Hilary Humphreys

Case history

A 4-year-old girl is brought to the Emergency Department (ED) by her parents and is admitted with a three-day history of cough, coryza, and mild conjunctivitis. She has a background history of T-cell lymphoma for which she is being treated. Her parents are not sure if she received both doses of the measles, mumps, and rubella (MMR) vaccine but otherwise her vaccinations are up to date. On examination, she has a temperature of 39 °C and has an extensive rash, mainly confined to the trunk, where there are defined areas of discolouration but no papules or macules. The rest of the physical examination is normal.

Questions

4.1 What is the differential diagnosis and how would you investigate this child?

4.2 What are the principles of the management of this child's condition?

4.3 How should spread be prevented or minimized, especially in healthcare institutions?

4.4 Are healthcare workers at increased risk of acquiring this condition?

Answers

4.1 What is the differential diagnosis and how would you investigate this child?

The presence of a rash and fever in a child represents an exanthema. These usually also involve the mucous membranes and are caused by a variety of viruses, the most common of which are:

- Varicella-zoster (VZ), parvovirus B19, enteroviruses, human herpes virus-6, measles, and rubella.
- If contracted abroad—chikungunya virus, dengue, and zika virus.

Diagnosis requires an accurate history, especially of immunizations and travel, examination, for example, is the rash vesicular—suggesting VZV or possibly enterovirus infection—or maculopapular, with laboratory testing of appropriate samples by serology and/or genome detection. A diagnosis of chickenpox (Case 3 'Chickenpox') is often made on clinical grounds, but can be confirmed by demonstration of VZV DNA in a vesicle swab. Demonstration of parvovirus IgM (immunoglobulin M) and a high viral load confirms acute parvovirus infection. Detection of enteroviral RNA in a vesicle swab, or, if there are no vesicles, a throat swab or faeces sample, suggests enterovirus infection; serology is unreliable. Detection of IgM antibodies or measles RNA in an oral swab is the most efficient way of diagnosing measles. Laboratory confirmation of measles is essential as the positive predictive value of a clinical diagnosis is poor, given the wide range of other conditions that can present with a maculopapular rash.

In an immunosuppressed child, the measles rash may be atypical as in the case described above and may not mimic that of the classical papular-purpuric rash (see Fig. 4.1). Children with defective cell-mediated immunity often develop an atypical rash and those born of human immunodeficiency virus (HIV)-positive mothers have lower concentrations of maternal antibodies with an increased susceptibility at a younger age. The combination of a prodromal illness with a cough, coryza, and conjunctivitis is very suggestive of measles and the presence of Koplik's spots (Fig. 4.2) is almost pathognomonic.

4.2 What are the principles of the management of this child's condition?

There is no specific antiviral therapy although agents such as ribavirin and interferon alpha have been used to treat central nervous system infections. The management approach is largely symptomatic, that is, fluids and paracetamol. However, vitamin A can reduce morbidity and mortality and the World Health Organization (WHO) recommends once-daily doses for two consecutive days to all children with measles who are twelve months or older. The main emphasis should also be on preventing onward spread.

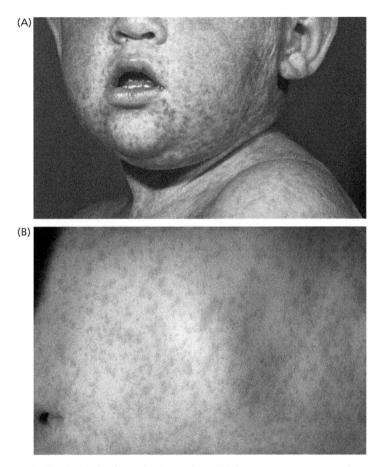

Figure 4.1 Classical rash of measles (see colour plate).

(A) Reproduced from CDC. ID#: 1150. 1963. https://phil.cdc.gov/details.aspx?pid=1150; (B) Reproduced from CDC/Heinz F. Eichenwald, MD. ID#3168. 1958. https://phil.cdc.gov/details.aspx?pid=3168.

4.3 How should spread be prevented or minimized, especially in healthcare institutions?

Measures should involve administrative controls, that is, measles vaccination, environmental controls such as placing a patient in a negative pressure ventilation room, and personal protective measures such as the use of FFP3 respiratory masks, or their equivalent. However, measles is highly infectious and is spread by the droplet route and patients should be isolated upon suspicion. Non-vaccinated exposed contacts should be vaccinated and in some instances normal human immunoglobulin should be administered, especially if they are immunocompromised or pregnant.

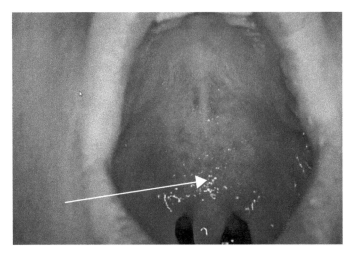

Figure 4.2 Koplik's spots on the buccal mucosa are highly suggestive of measles (see colour plate).

Reproduced from CDC/ Heinz F. Eichenwald, MD, 1958, https://phil.cdc.gov/Details.aspx?pid=3187.

4.4 Are healthcare workers at increased risk of acquiring this condition?

Yes. It has been estimated that healthcare workers have up to an 18-fold increased chance of acquiring measles compared with other adults in the community. This may arise from either not being vaccinated, having only received one dose of the vaccine, or from vaccine failure. Also, most healthcare workers would have been vaccinated many years earlier and the protective impact of the vaccine may have waned. In general, two doses of measles vaccine will provide long-lasting immunity.

Case history continued

A diagnosis of measles is confirmed by PCR of mouth washings. The patient is conservatively managed in hospital for two days and is subsequently discharged. She makes an uneventful recovery but six weeks later presents with confusion and ataxia, requiring neurological assessment.

Questions

4.5 What are the complications of measles?

4.6 What categories of encephalitis may arise following measles infection?

4.7 Has there been any major change in measles epidemiology in the United Kingdom and beyond in recent years?

Answers

4.5 What are the complications of measles?

Pneumonia, otitis media, and encephalitis are the most common complications. In resource-poor countries, many children with measles develop diarrhoea which contributes to undernutrition and they then often die of pneumonia. Complications are understandably more common and severe in immunocompromised patients.

4.6 What categories of encephalitis may arise following measles infection?

These are outlined in Table 4.1 and include primarily at the time of presentation or shortly afterwards, acute post-infectious measles encephalomyelitis, inclusion body encephalitis, and sub-acute sclerosing panencephalitis (SSPE). The case described is most likely to be acute post-infectious encephalitis.

Table 4.1 Categories of encephalitis associated with measles

	Primary	**Acute post-infectious**	**Inclusion body**	***SSPE**
Onset	At presentation	Weeks to months later	Within 1 year of infection or vaccination	Up to 20 years later after measles infection
Features	Signs and symptoms of encephalitis	Weakness and sensory loss	Seizures, altered mental state	Dementia and behaviour problems
Laboratory diagnosis	PCR, + ve	PCR +/–ve	PCR –ve but CSF antibodies elevated	PCR –ve but CSF antibodies very elevated
Outcome	10–15% die, 25% with neurological deficits, e.g. seizures	May fully recover and prognosis better than with primary encephalitis	75% die as often associated with immunosuppressive illness	Most die within 1–3 years after SSPE symptoms develop

*Sub-acute sclerosing panencephalitis

4.7 Has there been any major change in measles epidemiology in the United Kingdom and beyond in recent years?

Over the last 10 years there has been an increase in measles in many countries including the United Kingdom, after a period when the prevalence of measles was relatively low. This has arisen due to inadequate vaccination including the absence of a second dose of vaccine administered to children. Globally, measles remains one of the leading causes of death amongst children less than 5 years of age and in the WHO region for Europe, sporadic cases and outbreaks occur especially in countries with inadequate public health infrastructure. In particular, there is a need to verify vaccination rates in some countries and to acknowledge the susceptibility of some healthcare workers to measles. From the late 1990s to 2005, there was a 60% reduction in global mortality from over 800,000 to approximately 350,000. All the WHO regions have signed up to eliminate measles by 2020, but it remains to be seen whether this can be achieved.

Further reading

Buchanan R, Bonthius DJ. Measles virus and associated central nervous system sequelae. *Sem Pediatric Neurol* 2012; **19**: 107–14.

Keighley CL, Saunderson RB, Koh J, Dwyer E. Viral exanthems. *Curr Opin Infect Dis* 2015; **28**: 139–50.

Maltezou, HC, Wicker S. Measles in health-care settings. *Am J Infect Control* 2013; **41**: 661–3.

Moss WJ, Griffin DE. Measles. *Lancet* 2012; **379**: 153–64.

O'Connor P, Jankovic D, Muscat M, Ben-Mamou M, Reef S, et al. Measles and rubella elimination in the WHO Region for Europe: progress and challenges. *Clin Microbiol Infect* 2017; **23**: 504–10.

Case 5

Hilary Humphreys

Case history

A 25-year-old female goes to see her General Practitioner (GP) complaining of erythematous skin lesions on her back and abdomen that have been increasing in size (Fig. 5.1). She has described the lesions as expanding over the past two weeks but there is no temperature. She is a mechanical engineer and does a lot of cross-country walking in her leisure time. She is commenced on antimicrobial therapy.

Questions

5.1 What are the possible diagnoses here?

5.2 How does the aetiology and epidemiology of this infection in Europe and in the United Kingdom differ to that in North America?

5.3 How may a diagnosis of this infection be confirmed?

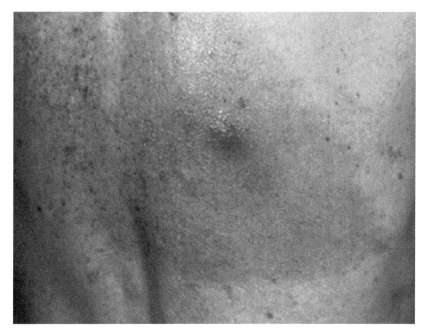

Figure 5.1 Skin lesion on back (see colour plate).

Reproduced with permission from Wormser GP, et al. (2010) Lyme borreliosis. In Warell DA, et al. (eds) *Oxford Textbook of Medicine, Fifth Edition*. Oxford: Oxford University Press.

Answers

5.1 What are the possible diagnoses here?

The appearance is strongly suggestive of erythema migrans, characteristic of infection due to *Borrelia* spp., the microbial cause of Lyme disease, which is a tick-borne infection. Other possibilities in the differential diagnosis are cellulitis but the patient has no temperature, contact dermatitis if there is an appropriate history, herpes simplex, or varicella-zoster infection, but these infections are usually characterized by vesicles, or finally fungal skin infection, but there is no scaling to suggest this.

5.2 How does the aetiology and epidemiology of this infection in Europe and in the United Kingdom differ to that in North America?

Approximately 4 out of 5 patients in the United States with erythema migrans have systemic symptoms such as malaise, headache, fever, and chills, as well as both myalgia and arthralgia. This systemic component is uncommon in the United Kingdom and Europe and may be attributable to the lower virulence of *B. afzelii*, the major cause in Europe compared with *B. burgdorferi sensu stricto*, the only species causing disease in the United States. *Ixodes ricinus*, a hard-bodied tick is the most common vector in the United Kingdom and Europe, in contrast to the United States where *I. scapularis* is the commonest with *I. pacificus* predominating on the west coast. Most cases in the United Kingdom occur between July and October. The condition is particularly common in the southern counties of England, but approximately 18% of cases in the United Kingdom are acquired abroad.

5.3 How may a diagnosis of this infection be confirmed?

Most cases of Lyme disease are routinely diagnosed by serology using a two-step approach, that is, enzyme immuno-assay (EIA), followed by Western blot. The Western blot is required to exclude cross-reaction antibodies in the EIA. However, EIAs based upon the C6 peptide are said to be more specific in diagnosis. If positive with these assays, this may suggest disease-acquired in Europe. Molecular methods such as PCR can be used on skin biopsies, blood samples, or sterile fluids, such as synovial or cerebrospinal fluid. In practice, PCR is mainly used for detecting Lyme arthritis. Culture of skin, fluid, and tissue is confined to specialist or research centres as it is technically demanding and requires the use of specialist media, and culture assessment with dark-field or fluorescent microscopy.

Case history continued

Lyme disease manifesting as erythema migrans is initially suspected and subsequently confirmed by EIA and Western blot. When she hears about the likely method of transmission, she asks how it might be prevented and whether the infection can become chronic.

Questions

5.4 What options are there for the treatment of Lyme disease?

5.5 What strategies are employed to minimize acquisition of Lyme disease?

5.6 What are the other manifestations of Lyme disease other than erythema migrans?

5.7 What are the features of chronic Lyme disease?

Answers

5.4 What options are there for the treatment of Lyme disease?

B. burgdorferii is susceptible to a range of antibiotics. However, for erythema migrans, doxycycline, amoxicillin, or cefuroxime axetil are the recommended drugs of choice (Table 5.1). Macrolides are considered to be second-line agents but the consensus is that for uncomplicated Lyme disease, 10 days of doxycycline is considered highly effective. Treatment of the central nervous system (CNS) manifestations includes ceftriaxone or doxycycline.

5.5 What strategies are employed to minimize acquisition of Lyme disease?

There are a number of approaches which include the following:

◆ Ticks, the vectors, are associated with specific habitats and where possible these should be avoided—mixed wooded areas that support rodents, birds, and deer.

◆ As there is an interval between the ticks starting to feed and being capable of transmitting the bacterium, inspecting the skin and removing ticks after exposure, such as after a walk or showering, will minimize the risk.

◆ The use of topical insect repellents, wearing long trousers, socks, and long shirts when in an endemic area and even clothing treated with permethrin, have all been suggested.

◆ Antibiotic prophylaxis has been suggested but is rarely indicated. It should be reserved for situations where there is a high risk of transmission, that is, where the tick has been attached for 36 hours.

Table 5.1 Treatment options for Lyme Disease

Condition	Antimicrobial options
Erythema migrans	Doxycycline × 10–14 days Alternatively, amoxicillin, cefuroxime axetil
Lyme meningitis	Doxycycline × 14 days Ceftriaxone × 14 days
Lyme arthritis	Doxycycline × 28 days
Lyme cardiac disease	Doxycycline × 14 days Alternatively, ceftriaxone followed by doxycycline × 14–21 days in total

Source: data from Sanchez E, Vannier E, Wormser GP and Hu LT. (2016). Diagnosis, treatment and prevention of Lyme disease, human granulocytic anaplasmosis, and babesiosis. *JAMA*. 315(16):1767–77. DOI:10.1001/jama.2016.2884.

5.6 What are the other manifestations of Lyme disease other than erythema migrans?

Lyme disease is a systemic infection and many organs or systems can be affected. Weeks, months or years after the initial contact with the responsible pathogen, neurological, cardiac, or musculoskeletal manifestations may occur. Meningitis, cranial nerve palsies, and mononeuritis multiplex are well-recognized presentations, and about one in ten of all patients with Lyme disease present with neurological manifestations. Cardiac involvement includes atrioventricular block, myocarditis, and possibly a form of cardiomyopathy. Arthritis may involve one or more joints with the knees or ankles most commonly affected.

5.7 What are the features of chronic Lyme disease?

This is a controversial clinical entity as a variety of symptoms have been attributed to either infection with *B. burgdorferi* or its subsequent complications. Many patients investigated for supposed chronic Lyme disease have no evidence of ever having had previous Lyme disease and the biomedical scientific community is not convinced about chronic infection as a clinical entity. However, many patients and advocacy groups believe that it exists and request investigation and treatment. It is important to exclude other potential causes of symptoms such as malaise, tiredness, and arthralgia, by excluding osteoarthritis, rheumatoid arthritis, and other connective tissue diseases. There is little evidence to suggest that ongoing symptoms after antibiotic treatment for Lyme disease are due to persistent infection.

Acknowledgement

With thanks to Dr Sinéad O'Donnell.

Further reading

Baker PJ, Wormser GP. The clinical relevance of studies on *Borrelia burgdorferi* persisters. *Am J Med* 2017; **130**: 1009–10.

Dubrey SW, Bhatia A, Woodham S, Rakowicz W. Lyme disease in the United Kingdom. *Postgrad Med J* 2014; **90**: 33–42.

Nadelman RB. Erythema migrans. *Infect Dis Clin North Am* 2015; **29**: 211–39.

NICE (National Institute for Health and Care Excellence). Lyme disease (NG95). 2018. http://www.nice.org.uk/guidance/ng95 accessed 21 July 2019.

Sanchez E, Vannier E, Wormser GP, Hu LT. Diagnosis, treatment and prevention of Lyme disease, human granulocytic anaplasmosis, and babesiosis. *J Am Med Assoc* 2016; **315**: 1767–77.

Section 2

Respiratory tract

Case 6 – Case 14

Case 6

Maheshi Ramasamy

Case history

A previously fit and well 67-year-old man presents to his General Practitioner (GP) with a 4-day history of cough, myalgia, and breathlessness. On examination he is febrile but oriented. His pulse rate is 110/minute, his blood pressure is 95/60, and his respiration rate is 25/minute. He has coarse crackles on auscultation of his R lung base. The GP considers a diagnosis of community-acquired pneumonia (CAP). The patient has lived in the United Kingdom all his life and has never been abroad. He has no unwell contacts, works in a supermarket, and his only pets are goldfish.

Questions

6.1 Should this patient be managed in the community or admitted to hospital?

6.2 What initial non-microbiological investigations should be performed in hospital?

6.3 What specimens need to be taken for microbiology assessment?

6.4 What is the role of urinary pneumococcal antigen testing?

6.5 What is role of PCR and serology?

6.6 Is routine antibiotic coverage for atypical organisms (e.g. a macrolide or quinolone) required in this patient?

Answers

6.1 Should this patient be managed in the community or admitted to hospital?

The CRB-65 score (**C**onfusion, **R**espiratory rate, **B**lood pressure, age **65** or over) enables rapid assessment of severity and guides the initial decision about management in the community. For patients assessed in hospital, this is modified to the CURB-65 score to include **U**rea (Fig. 6.1). The CURB-65 score should be used in conjunction with clinical judgement. This patient has a score of 2 and hospital-based care should be considered. The CURB-65 score has not been validated for immunocompromised patients, and care should be taken in assessing these patients who can rapidly progress from mild to severe illness.

6.2 What initial non-microbiological investigations should be performed in hospital?

Routine investigations are not recommended for mild cases of pneumonia managed in the community. For patients assessed in hospital, chest X-ray (CXR) should be performed to look for infiltrates or complications of pneumonia such as a pleural effusion or cavitation. Routine bloods including full blood count, serum biochemistry, liver function tests, C-reactive protein, and pulse oximetry should also be performed.

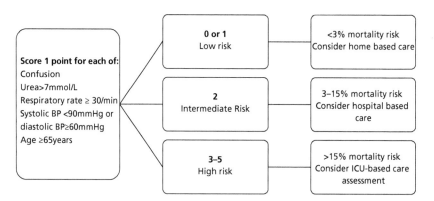

Figure 6.1 CURB-65 severity scoring system for community-acquired pneumonia.

Adapted with permission from Lim WS, et al. (2009). Pneumonia Guidelines Committee of the BTS Standards of Care Committee. BTS Guidelines for the management of community acquired pneumonia in adults: update. *Thorax.* 64(Suppl 3):1–55. DOI: http://dx.doi.org/10.1136/thx.2009.121434.

6.3 What specimens need to be taken for microbiology assessment?

The most common cause of CAP is adults in *Streptococcus pneumoniae* (Table 6.1) and current guidelines recommend empiric regimens that cover this organism. Blood cultures are only positive in 5–15% of patients with CAP. Patients with severe CAP are more likely to have an alternative causative organism to *S. pneumoniae*, such as *Staphylococcus aureus, Legionella* spp., or Gram-negative bacilli. Blood cultures should be obtained in all cases of severe CAP to detect organisms not covered by empiric antibiotic regimens. The value of sputum cultures in CAP is limited as they are contaminated with upper respiratory tract flora. Yield is dependent on the quality of collection and specimen handling. Endotracheal aspirates and broncho-alveolar lavage (BAL) sampling are more representative of lower respiratory tract flora, less likely to be contaminated with oropharyngeal commensals but are only possible if the patient requires ventilation. When suspected, culture of respiratory samples for *Legionella* spp. should be requested. The collection of samples for bacteriological culture should where possible be carried out before the administration of antimicrobials in order to increase the likelihood of a microbiological diagnosis but initiation of treatment should not be delayed for this purpose. A virology throat

Table 6.1 Common aetiologies of community-acquired pneumonia

Severity of CAP	Likely aetiology
Mild	*Streptococcus pneumoniae*
	Mycoplasma pneumoniae
	Haemophilus influenzae
	Chlamydophila pneumoniae/psittaci
	Influenza and other respiratory viruses
Moderate	*S. pneumoniae*
	M. pneumoniae
	Chlamydophila spp.
	H. influenzae
	Legionella spp.
	Aspiration
	Influenza and other respiratory viruses
Severe	*S. pneumoniae*
	Staphylococcus aureus
	Legionella spp.
	Gram-negative bacilli
	H. influenzae
	Influenza

Source: data from Lim WS, et al. (2009). Pneumonia Guidelines Committee of the BTS Standards of Care Committee. BTS Guidelines for the management of community acquired pneumonia in adults: update 2009. *Thorax*. 64(Suppl 3):1–55. DOI: http://dx.doi.org/10.1136/thx.2009.121434.

swab for polymerase chain reaction (PCR) detection of respiratory viruses should be considered (see Question 5).

In selected patients with risk factors (immunosuppression) and compatible clinical features, *Pneumocystis jirovecii* infection should be considered. Samples such as induced sputum or broncho-alveolar lavage should be obtained for cytological and/ or molecular detection methods.

6.4 What is the role of urinary pneumococcal antigen testing?

Urinary antigen tests are available for pneumococcal detection with a sensitivity of between 50% and 80% and specificity of approximately 90%. This has the advantage of being quick in the setting where microbiological samples are not available for diagnosis and may allow earlier rationalization of antibiotics. Urine antigen is detectable in 83% of individuals even after 3 days of antibiotics. Urine legionella antigen tests only detect *L. pneumophila* serogroup 1, which is responsible for 80–95% of all legionella cases. The sensitivity is 70–90% and the specificity 99% for *L. pneumophila* type 1. Urinary antigen is positive from the first day of symptoms and can remain positive for weeks.

6.5 What is the role of PCR and serology?

Molecular diagnostics—that is, multiplex PCR for respiratory viruses (influenza A and B, parainfluenza 1–3, adenovirus, respiratory syncytial virus)—can be considered in severe cases, in outbreaks, and in immunocompromised or pregnant patients. This can be done on respiratory samples, for example, a virology throat swab, a sputum sample, or lower respiratory tract samples. In some cases (e.g. outbreaks) molecular diagnostics for atypical pathogens such as *Mycoplasma pneumoniae* or *Chlamydophila* spp. may be considered.

Serological diagnosis of *M. pneumoniae* and *Chlamydophila* spp. and *Legionella* spp. requires comparison of acute and convalescent phase-specific antibody titres. Antibiotic therapy is usually complete by the earliest sampling time for convalescent titres, and therefore serology adds little value to the acute diagnosis of CAP except in the epidemiological investigation of outbreaks.

6.6 Is routine antibiotic coverage for atypical organisms (e.g. a macrolide or quinolone) required in this patient?

'Atypical' pneumonia tends to occur in epidemics, in otherwise healthy individuals, and is caused by intracellular organisms that do not respond to β-lactam agents such as *Legionella* spp., *M. pneumoniae*, or *Chlamydophila* spp. The British Thoracic Society guidelines (Table 6.2) recommend β-lactam monotherapy in mild cases of CAP, when disease is likely to be caused by a susceptible pathogen such as

Table 6.2 Antibiotic therapy for CAP

Pneumonia severity	First line	Alternative(s)
Mild *Treat for 3–5 days*	An oral penicillin e.g. amoxicillin 500 mg tds	Oral macrolide e.g. clarithromycin 500 mg bd OR Oral tetracycline e.g. doxycycline 100mg od
Moderate *Consider treating for 7–10 days*	An oral/intravenous penicillin e.g. amoxicillin 500 mg tds po/iv PLUS oral/intravenous macrolide e.g. clarithromycin 500 mg bd po/iv	Oral respiratory quinolone e.g. moxifloxacin 400 mg od OR Oral tetracycline e.g. doxycycline 100 mg od
Severe *Consider treating for 7–10 days*	Intravenous broad spectrum pencillin e.g. co-amoxiclav 1.2 g tds iv PLUS po/iv macrolide e.g. clarithromycin 500 mg bd po/iv	Intravenous cephalosporin e.g. ceftriaxone 2 g od iv PLUS oral/intravenous macrolide e.g. clarithromycin 500 mg bd po/iv

Source: data from Lim WS, et al. (2009). Pneumonia Guidelines Committee of the BTS Standards of Care Committee. BTS Guidelines for the management of community acquired pneumonia in adults: update 2009. *Thorax.* 64(Suppl 3):1–55. DOI: http://dx.doi.org/10.1136/thx.2009.121434.

S. pneumoniae. Mild *M. pneumoniae* or *Chlamydophila* infections usually resolve without pathogen-directed therapy. Failure to respond to first-line antibiotics should, however, prompt investigation for *Legionella* spp. or penicillin-resistant pneumococcal infection. In more severe cases of CAP, or in those where an atypical pathogen is strongly suspected, a macrolide or a respiratory quinolone should be included. The Infectious Diseases Society of America/American Thoracic Society guidelines recommend a respiratory quinolone or β-lactam/macrolide combination therapy for mild CAP, but this reflects the higher incidence of penicillin-resistant *S. pneumoniae* in North America. This patient does not therefore require atypical coverage on epidemiological grounds.

Further reading

Lim WS, Badouin SV, George RC, Hill AT, Jamieson C, et al. Pneumonia Guidelines Committee of the BTS Standards of Care Committee. BTS Guidelines for the management of community acquired pneumonia in adults: update. *Thorax* 2009; **64**: 1–55.

Mandell LA, Wunderink RG, Anzueto A, Bartlett JG, Douglas Campbell G, et al. Infectious Diseases Society of America/American Thoracic Society Consensus Guidelines on the management of community acquired pneumonia in adults. *Clin Infec Dis* 2007; **44**: S27–72.

Mills GD, Oehley MR, Arrol B. Effectiveness of beta lactam antibiotics compared with antibiotics against atypical pathogens in non-severe community acquired pneumonia: meta-analysis. *Br Med J* 2005; **330**: 456.

Public Health England. Pneumonia. UK Standards for Microbiology Investigations. [Internet] London: PHE; 2014 [updated June 2014; cited August 2017]. Available at: http://www.hpa.org. uk/SMI/pdf.

Case 7

Hilary Humphreys

Case history

A 55-year-old man presents to the Emergency Department (ED) with increasing shortness of breath and cough. He is breathless with minimal exercise and although he has had a chronic cough, he has been expectorating purulent sputum for the last 3 days. He has a background history of ischaemic heart disease for which he underwent stenting 3 years previously. He works as a car mechanic and has a history of smoking more than 40 pack years. On examination, his vital signs are normal, he has some wheeze on forced exhalation and there is evidence of hyperinflation as revealed by increased resonance on percussion.

Questions

7.1 What is the diagnosis?

7.2 What is the role of sputum and other microbiological investigations?

7.3 What antimicrobial agents are indicated?

7.4 What is the role of the normal flora in this condition?

7.5 What is the role for prophylactic antibiotics in patients with this condition?

Answers

7.1 What is the diagnosis?

Given the history, it is likely that this patient has chronic obstructive pulmonary disease (COPD) and that he is presenting with an acute exacerbation. Chronic bronchitis is the commonest form of COPD and is characterized by a productive cough for 3 months in each of the 2 previous successive years, but in a stable patient, this is often minimal and mucoid in nature. The onset of increased sputum production and a change from mucoid to purulent is typical of an acute exacerbation. In advanced COPD, the chest X-ray (CXR) and computerized tomography (CT) scan may show evidence of hyperinflation such as a flat diaphragm and increased radiolucency without any obvious abnormalities in acute exacerbations, specifically opacification suggestive of infection. However, it is important to exclude pneumonia on physical examination and by CXR (Fig. 7.1).

7.2 What is the role of sputum and other microbiological investigations?

The value of sending sputum for microscopy and culture in this setting is controversial but probably has little or no value once antibiotics have been started. In primary care, sputum is not indicated, samples are often of poor quality, and the results often reflect colonizing flora. Sputum culture in a patient presenting to

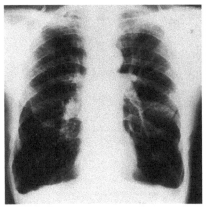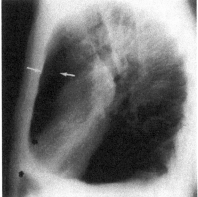

Figure 7.1 Posterior anterior and lateral chest X-ray showing typical features in a patient with COPD, i.e. low and flat diaphragm (black arrows), obtuse costo-phrenic angles and retro-sternal transradiency (white arrows).

Table 7.1 Microbial causes of acute exacerbations of COPD

Microbe	Frequency	Comment
Bacteria		
Haemophilus influenzae	Common	Major pathogen
Streptococcus pneumoniae	Common	Major pathogen
Moraxella catarrhalis	Less common	Minor pathogen
Pseudomonas aeruginosa	Less common	Important in advanced disease +/– bronchiectasis
Staphylococcus aureus	Uncommon	Minor pathogen
Viruses		
Rhinovirus	Common	Minor role in stable disease
Respiratory syncytial virus	Less common	Often only detected by molecular methods
Metapneumovirus	Increasingly recognised	Often only confirmed by molecular techniques
Influenza	Less common	Seasonal importance
Others		
Chlamydophila pneumoniae	Uncommon	Significance uncertain
Pneumocystis jiroveci	Uncommon/rare	Significance uncertain

hospital with increasingly purulent sputum and who is not on antibiotics may be helpful. Blood cultures are not indicated as there is no fever, nor are urinary legionella and pneumococcal antigen in the absence of evidence of pneumonia. Acute exacerbations of COPD can be caused by viruses, but often no microbial cause is identified. Table 7.1 outlines some of the more important causes and their potential significance. If there is a microbial aetiology, confirmation will depend on recent treatment with antimicrobial agents and the extent of investigations. Molecular detection methods are increasingly identifying viral and other causes such as influenza, para-influenza, metapneumovirus, and respiratory syncytial virus, as well as *Chlamydophila pneumoniae*.

7.3 What antimicrobial agents are indicated?

In patients with an acute exacerbation of COPD with purulent sputum, antibiotics are generally prescribed even if the evidence for this is considered poor. The rationale for this is that antibiotics reduce the bacterial load and therefore help minimize the inflammatory response, which is very much part of the pathology of

COPD, particularly during exacerbations. Therefore, consider prescribing an antibiotic if the symptoms are severe, and the sputum is purulent. In apyrexial patients with no change in sputum, antibiotics may be withheld. The choice of antibiotic will be governed by whether the patient has recently been on antibiotics, the likely pathogens or what is detected, and local resistance patterns. Initial treatment may include an agent like co-amoxiclav, which will cover most of the likely bacterial pathogens. Macrolides will treat chlamydophila but in patients with heart disease, caution should be exercised as macrolides prolong the QTc interval. *Pseudomonas aeruginosa* is occasionally isolated, especially in patients with co-existent bronchiectasis, in which case an agent with anti-pseudomonal activity such as piperacillin/tazobactam may be indicated.

7.4 What is the role of the normal flora in this condition?

There is now much interest in the microbiome of the respiratory tract and its contribution to chronic lung diseases, both when the condition is stable and during exacerbations. Recent studies have shown an unprecedented complexity of the respiratory microbiota during exacerbations with a wide array of phylogenetically distinct bacteria, far more than previously recognized from exclusively culture-based studies. The diversity of colonizing bacteria outside of acute exacerbations appears to be much less. With COPD there are alterations in the bacterial growth conditions, resulting in greater bacterial diversity with increased airways inflammation, resulting in acute exacerbations of COPD. However, longitudinal studies are required to determine variations over time and any correlations with measures of inflammation.

7.5 What is the role for prophylactic antibiotics in patients with this condition?

This is a controversial area in medical practice. The rationale is analogous to the use of prophylactic antibiotics in patients with cystic fibrosis to prevent acute exacerbations or chronic carriage of certain pathogens. A number of studies suggest that long-term oral antibiotic treatment in COPD and patients with bronchiectasis reduces exacerbation frequency and may have immunomodulatory effects. Macrolides such as azithromycin reduce the concentrations of pro-inflammatory cytokines, influence toll-like receptors, and enhance phagocytosis, thus limiting the inflammatory response. However, this has to be balanced by the risks of antibiotic resistance and the side effectsof such antibiotics. The United Kingdom National Institute for Health and Care Excellence (NICE) guidelines on COPD suggest that prophylactic antibiotics may be given if one or more of the following apply:

♦ Frequent exacerbations with sputum production

♦ Prolonged exacerbations

♦ Exacerbations requiring hospitalization

The NICE guidelines recommend first confirming the absence of a prolonged QT interval and baseline liver function tests before starting the prophylaxis. Also, the possible side effects of azithromycin should be fully discussed with the patient. Therefore, this approach is reserved for some patients with COPD but the azithromycin should be continued when other antibiotics are given to treat COPD exacerbations. This approach and other factors have stimulated increasing interest in the inflammatory response in COPD and whether cytokines influence presentation and outcome.

Further reading

Chen Y-W R, Leung JM, Sin DD. A systematic review of diagnostic biomarkers of COPD exacerbation. *PLoS One* 2016; **11**: eD158843. doi: 10.1371/journal.pone.0158843.

Dickson RP, Martinez FJ, Huffnagle GB. The role of the microbiome in exacerbations of chronic lung di*seases. Lancet* 2014; **384**: 691–702.

Hopkinson NS, Molyneux A, Pink J, Harrisingh MC, on behalf of the Guideline Committee. Chronic obstructive pulmonary disease: diagnosis and management: summary of updated NICE guidance. *Br Med J* 2019; **366**: I4486. doi:10.1136/bmj.I4486.

Santos S, Marin A, Serra-Batlles J, de al Rosa D, Solanes I, et al. Treatment of patients with COPD and recurrent exacerbations: the role of infection and inflammation. *Inter J COPD* 2016; **11**: 515–25.

Zwaans WAR, Mallia P, van Winden MEC, Rohde GGU. The relevance of respiratory viral infections in the exacerbations of chronic obstructive pulmonary disease—a systematic review. *J Clin Vir* 2014; **61**:181–8.

Case 8

Hilary Humphreys

Case history

A 25-year-old female, who is 35 weeks pregnant, is referred to the Emergency Department (ED) in mid-January. She has a 2-day history of a non-productive cough, she is feeling feverish, and she complains of tiredness and anorexia. She has no relevant previous medical history and is on no medications. On examination, she has a temperature of 38.5 °C but otherwise the rest of the physical examination is unremarkable. She is admitted for observation and investigation for probable influenza.

Questions

8.1 What complications may arise from influenza during pregnancy?

8.2 Should this patient receive antiviral treatment?

8.3 What categories of patients should be treated for influenza or receive prophylaxis if exposed?

Answers

8.1 What complications may arise from influenza during pregnancy?

Pregnant women with influenza are at increased risk of cardio-respiratory complications and the need for admission to the intensive care unit (ICU). These risks are further exacerbated by underlying diseases such as diabetes mellitus. This virus infection can result in miscarriage, small-for-gestational age, and the need for admission to the neonatal ICU.

8.2 Should this patient receive antiviral treatment?

Yes. The current treatment of influenza is with a neuraminidase inhibitor, that is, oral oseltamivir. Alternatives, especially in the ICU, include inhaled zanamivir and intravenous zanamivir or IV peramivir. Baloxivir is a new oral antiviral treatment for influenza that inhibits cap-dependent endonuclease and may be an alternative in the future.

In the context of a pregnant patient, there is a balance to be made between the need to treat the mother aggressively, given the increased risk of complications, and the potential risks to the foetus from treatment with the most likely agent, oseltamivir. Antiviral treatment can lessen the symptoms, shorten the length of the disease, and reduce the risk of perinatal complications. To date, there has been no convincing evidence of adverse consequences to the foetus from oseltamivir and therefore this antiviral treatment should be administered.

Zanamivir is considered when there is suspected poor gastrointestinal absorption or failure to respond to oseltamivir (suspected resistance). Zanamivir should be avoided in pregnancy unless the expected benefit outweighs the danger to the foetus. There are no safety data on peramivir in pregnancy.

8.3 What categories of patients should be treated for influenza or receive prophylaxis if exposed?

Previously healthy individuals do not usually require antiviral treatment. However, in addition to pregnant women, those who are severely immunosuppressed, those who have chronic respiratory, cardiovascular, liver, renal, and endocrine disease, and those ill enough to require acute admission to hospital, should be treated for influenza or receive prophylaxis if exposed to influenza but who are not yet symptomatic.

Case history continued

The patient is started on oseltamivir but 48 hours later requires admission to the ICU because of increasing respiratory distress. Genome amplification by RT-PCR (reverse transcription PCR) of a nasopharyngeal swab is positive for influenza A H3N2, and other investigations are normal. Follow-up CXR from that done on admission to the ICU shows infiltrations in the left-mid zone. She requires intubation and ventilation. Three new cases of influenza-like illness are reported on the ward where this patient was originally admitted. These patients had been in-patients for over 7 days and therefore these are cases of hospital-acquired influenza.

Questions

8.4   What is the most likely infective pulmonary complication associated with influenza?

8.5   What factors contribute to outbreaks of nosocomial influenza?

8.6   Why are uptake rates for influenza vaccines so poor amongst healthcare professionals?

8.7   What categories of patients and others should be vaccinated annually against influenza?

8.8   How does avian influenza differ from seasonal influenza?

Answers

8.4 What is the most likely infective pulmonary complication associated with influenza?

Bacterial pneumonia is the most likely complication and this increases the mortality associated with influenza. The risk of bacterial super-infection is increased through virus-induced cytopathological damage and the overproduction of inflammatory cytokines, but it may take up to 21 days to present. *Streptococcus pneumoniae* is the most commonly identified cause followed by *Haemophilus influenzae* and *Staphylococcus aureus*. However, with the increasing use of molecular detection systems, including multiplex PCR, other viruses may be associated with influenza as co-pathogens such as respiratory syncytial virus and human metapneumovirus.

8.5 What factors contribute to outbreaks of nosocomial influenza?

These include:

- Low adherence to routine infection prevention and control measures (standard precautions)
- Delayed diagnosis
- Variable vaccine effectiveness
- Transmissibility of influenza with a reproductive number of 1–2, that is 1 to 2 other patients develop influenza if in contact with an index case, in the absence of isolation/cohorting
- Poor vaccine uptake amongst healthcare professionals (HCP)

This patient should have been isolated with respiratory precautions on admission. Measures to minimize the onward transmission of influenza in hospitals are outlined in Table 8.1.

8.6 Why are uptake rates for influenza vaccines so poor amongst healthcare professionals?

This is due to a number of reasons including fear that the vaccine will give the healthcare worker influenza (not true as it is a sub-unit and not a live vaccine), scepticism about the vaccine effectiveness, fear of side effects, and difficulty in accessing the vaccines either due to unavailability locally or in some countries the need to pay.

Table 8.1 Measures to prevent hospital-acquired influenza

Intervention	Comment
Effective surveillance	Monitor national and local trends including positive test results and reports of influenza-like illnesses
Early diagnosis	Same day testing: point-of-care testing may have a role in certain settings
Droplet precautions	Isolation on suspicion in the ED or on admission Surgical masks can reduce aerosol shedding
Antiviral prophylaxis	Administer to those exposed to known cases, especially if in a risk group for vaccination, e.g. elderly or chronic respiratory disease
Vaccination	Optimize·vaccination amongst the general population at the start of influenza season. Maximize healthcare professional vaccinations; in some countries it is mandatory

8.7 What categories of patients and others should be vaccinated annually against influenza?

In the United Kingdom, the categories of individuals who should be vaccinated are:

- All patients with chronic neurological, heart, renal, liver, and respiratory disease
- Pregnant mothers
- Patients with underlying immunosuppression
- Patients with diabetes mellitus
- Those who are morbidly obese, that is, with a body mass index of 40 or above
- Patients over 65 years of age
- Residents in long-stay residential homes
- All children aged 2–9 nine years of age
- Specifically, in pregnant women, influenza vaccination may reduce the likelihood of prematurity, smaller infant size at birth, and reduce the chances of the infant developing influenza during the first few months of life

8.8 How does avian influenza differ from seasonal influenza?

Avian influenza may be more pathogenic when it crosses the species barrier from birds to humans (Fig. 8.1). Human infection with avian H5N1 strains was first

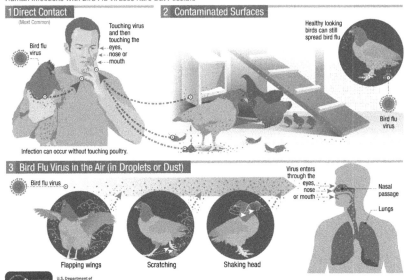

How Infected Backyard Poultry Could Spread Bird Flu to People
Human Infections with Bird Flu Viruses Rare But Possible

1 Direct Contact (Most Common)

Touching virus and then touching the eyes, nose or mouth

Bird flu virus

Infection can occur without touching poultry.

2 Contaminated Surfaces

Healthy looking birds can still spread bird flu

Bird flu virus

3 Bird Flu Virus in the Air (in Droplets or Dust)

Bird flu virus

Flapping wings   Scratching   Shaking head

Virus enters through the eyes, nose or mouth

Nasal passage

Lungs

U.S. Department of Health and Human Services
Centers for Disease Control and Prevention

www.cdc.gov/flu/avianflu/avian-in-humans.htm

Bird flu infections in people are rare, but possible. Most reported bird flu infections in people have happened after unprotected contact with infected birds or contaminated surfaces. This fact sheet has information about bird flu and bird flu infections in people.

Bird Flu in Birds

Wild water birds (like ducks and geese) can be infected with bird flu viruses, but usually do not get sick. Infected birds have virus in their saliva, mucous and droppings (feces). Bird flu viruses spread easily between birds. Some of these viruses can cause serious illness and death in domestic poultry (like chickens, ducks and turkeys).

Bird Flu & People

It is rare for people to get infected with bird flu viruses, but it can happen. Bird flu viruses can infect people when enough virus gets into a person's eyes, nose or mouth, or is inhaled. This might happen when virus is in the air (in droplets or possibly dust) and a person breathes it in, or when a person touches something that has virus on it and then touches their mouth, eyes or nose. (See picture on reverse side.) Most bird flu infections in people have happened after unprotected contact with infected birds or contaminated surfaces. In some cases, however, no direct contact has been reported. No human bird flu infections have been reported from proper handling of poultry meat or from eating properly cooked poultry or poultry products.

Bird flu illness in people has ranged from mild to severe. Signs and symptoms of bird flu infections in people can include: fever (temperature of 100°F [37.8°C] or greater) or feeling feverish, cough, sore throat, runny or stuffy nose, muscle or body aches, fatigue, headaches, eye redness (or conjunctivitis), and difficulty breathing. Other possible symptoms are diarrhea, nausea, and vomiting. As with seasonal flu, some people are at high risk of getting very sick from bird flu infections, including pregnant women, people with weakened immune systems and people 65 and older. Human infections with bird flu viruses usually can be treated with the same prescription drugs that are used to treat human seasonal flu viruses. These are called "flu antiviral drugs."

Bird Flu Outbreaks in Birds

Outbreaks of bird flu happen among birds from time to time. When deadly bird flu outbreaks happen in U.S. poultry, the United States Department of Agriculture (USDA) works with industry, state and other government partners to stop the outbreak so that it does not spread to other poultry. The Centers for Disease Control and Prevention works with partners to protect the public's health during these outbreaks. The risk to the public from bird flu outbreaks is low; however, because other bird flu viruses have infected people, it is possible that human infections with these viruses could occur. Risk depends on exposure. People with no contact with infected poultry or contaminated surfaces are thought to be at very low to no risk of infection. People with close or prolonged unprotected contact with infected birds or contaminated environments are thought to be at greater (though probably still low) risk of infection.

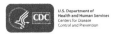

U.S. Department of Health and Human Services
Centers for Disease Control and Prevention

More information about bird flu is available at **www.cdc.gov/flu/avianflu**

Figure 8.1 Spread of avian influenza from birds to humans (see colour plate).

Reproduced from Center for Disease Control and Prevention (CDC). *Avian Influenza A Virus Infections in Human.* https://www.cdc.gov/flu/avianflu/avian-in-humans.htm.

described in Hong Kong in 1997. The strain has subsequently spread in avian species to other parts of Asia, Egypt, and occasionally to both North America and Europe. Direct exposure to infected birds may result in transmission to humans. Infection is often in a younger patient cohort than seasonal influenza and the case-fatality rate is around 50%. Ongoing surveillance, vaccination of poultry where feasible, and a high index of suspicion in patients with influenza-like illness recently returned from an area where it has been reported are all measures that can help reduce onward transmission both in the community and in hospitals. There are other avian strains such as H7N9 which also cause sporadic human infection with high mortality rates. There is also the potential of these strains evolving into pandemic strains through adaptive mutations within the human host, as may have been the origin of the 1918–19 strain.

Further reading

Ghulmiyyah LM, Alame MM, Mirza FG, Zaraket H, Nassar AH. Influenza and its treatment during pregnancy: a review. *J Neonatal-Perinatal Med* 2015; **8**: 297–306.

Joseph C, Togawa Y, Shindo N. Bacterial and viral infections associated with influenza. *Influen Other Resp Vir* 2013; 7: 105–13.

Lai S, Qin Y, Cowling BJ, et al. Global epidemiology of avian influenza A H5N1 virus infection in humans, 1997–2015: a systematic review of individual case data. *Lancet Infect Dis* 2016; 16: e108–18.

Public Health England guidance on the use of antiviral agents for the treatment and prophylaxis of seasonal influenza. Public Health England, October 2018. https://assets.publishing.service. gov.uk/government/uploads/system/uploads/attachment_data/file/761841/PHE_guidance_ antivirals_influenza_201819.pdf

Vanhems P, Bénet T, Munier-Marion E. Nosocomial influenza: encouraging insights and future challenges. *Curr Opin Infect Dis* 2016; **29**: 366–72.

Case 9

Nicola Jones

Case history

A 21-year-old male student presents to the Emergency Department (ED). He complains of chest pain, breathlessness, and cough. He is a Saudi national studying in England. He returned home for a family wedding and had spent 3 weeks staying with relatives in urban areas of Saudi Arabia, returning to the United Kingdom 6 days previously. He has a history of asthma, is on steroids and bronchodilator inhalers. He is a non-smoker.

He is febrile (38.5 °C) and has mild dyspnoea. Some crepitations are heard in the chest. A CT-pulmonary arteroiogram is negative for a pulmonary embolism but shows bilateral parenchymal shadowing consistent with a pneumonic process. The infiltrates are not in a lobar pattern, consistent with atypical infection.

Questions

9.1 What actions would you take in the immediate management of this case?

9.2 What are the differential diagnoses?

9.3 Does a history of travel suggest other infections?

9.4 What microbiology investigations should be organized?

9.5 A throat swab is positive for the presence of influenza virus. Does this change your management plan?

Answers

9.1 What actions would you take in the immediate management of this case?

The immediate concern is whether this patient fits the criteria for suspected Middle Eastern Respiratory Syndrome corona virus (MERS-CoV) infection. MERS-CoV represents a major infection control hazard to clinical staff and other patients. He should immediately be transferred to a single room with respiratory isolation. Ideally the isolation room should have an ante-room for donning and doffing of enhanced/high level personal protective equipment (PPE) and have negative pressure ventilation. A minimum number of trained staff (usually 2) caring for him should enter the room wearing PPE, which includes a full-face visor and face mask (FFP3) or respirator with hepafiltration (Fig. 9.1). A throat swab, sputum, or nasopharyngeal swabs should be taken for diagnosis. These samples are sent for rapid PCR-based testing for MERS-CoV. PPE should be worn by all staff entering the room until it is clear that MERS-CoV is not the cause of the pneumonia. Sputum- or aerosol-generating procedures (e.g. nebulizers) should not be performed with other unnecessary staff members present in the room.

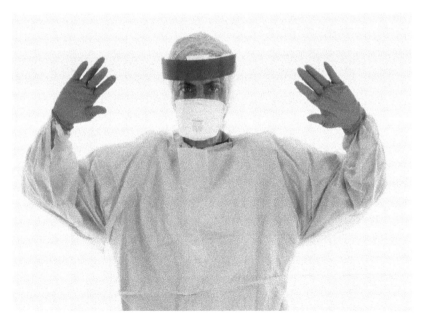

Figure 9.1 HCW wearing PPE for MERS-CoV.

Reproduced courtesy of Elham Khatamzas, Oxford University Hospitals NHS Foundation Trust, UK and TH Nicolas Wong, Buckinghamshire Healthcare NHS Trust, UK.

MERS-CoV is a highly pathogenic respiratory virus which currently is respon-sible for an epidemic of severe respiratory illness in the Arabian Peninsula. The virus, which is related to Severe Acute Respiratory Syndrome corona virus (SARS-CoV) and other corona viruses, is important as it may cause severe respiratory dis-tress associated with high mortality, and because of its ability to transmit to others, including in the nosocomial setting to healthcare workers and other patients by the respiratory route.

An epidemic of MERS-CoV occurred in South Korea in 2015. A single case brought the infection into South Korea from the Middle East. The diagnosis was not initially suspected in the index case and the resultant epidemic affected 186 people with 36% of cases being fatal. Twenty per cent of cases were healthcare workers.

9.2 What are the differential diagnoses?

The radiology findings have been described as 'atypical' by the radiologist. This means that the alveolar pattern of shadowing is more diffuse, widespread, and does not fall into a lobar distribution. Sometimes the term 'atypical' pneumonia is used to describe pneumonia accompanied by other features, such as deranged liver tests, renal function, and hyponatraemia.

In an immunocompetent host as here, the common bacterial causes of atypical pneumonia are *Legionella pneumophila*, *Mycoplasma pneumoniae*, and *Coxsiella burnetti* (Q fever). Respiratory viruses are also common and influenza, parainflu-enza, rhinovirus, metapneumovirus, and respiratory syncytial virus (RSV) can cause community-acquired pneumonia in healthy adults.

9.3 Does a history of travel suggest other infections?

Yes. Many respiratory pathogens have a global distribution, but others are more common in one geographical area. It is important to be aware of this global distri-bution when faced with a traveller from another region as the origin of their disease may reflect the country where they have travelled from rather than the one in which they present. Important viral respiratory pathogens that may be imported in to the United Kingdom are:

1. Avian Influenza A (H5 viruses) were first described in 1996 in poultry in China and has since spread rapidly in birds becoming endemic in poultry flocks in Bangladesh, China, Egypt, India, Indonesia, and Vietnam (see Case 8). Rare sporadic human cases have been seen in these countries, usually in those with contact with poultry and there has been minimal person-to-person transmis-sion. Disease in humans is often severe with high mortality.

2. Avian influenza A, H7N9, was first described in China in 2013 and since then has caused annual epidemics in humans there. Like H5N1, human disease tends to be a severe pneumonia and case fatality rates of 40% are seen. Thus far

1,558 human cases have been reported, usually in people with poultry exposure and acquisition of disease in mainland China. Cases are sporadic with limited person-to-person spread, but this virus is considered to have the greatest potential to cause a pandemic, as well as potentially posing the greatest risk of severely impacting on public health.

Most of the cases of human infection with avian H7N9 virus have reported recent exposure to live poultry or potentially contaminated environments, especially markets where live birds have been sold. This virus does not appear to transmit easily from person to person, and sustained human-to-human transmission has not been reported.

3. *Hantavirus pulmonary syndrome* (HPS, e.g. sin nombre virus) causes severe respiratory distress following airborne exposure to rodents or their droppings, specifically work-related exposure, camping and hiking, house or out-building cleaning. Typically, HPS is acquired in North America (west of the Mississippi River) and Latin America.

4. *Severe Acute Respiratory Syndrome corona virus* (SARS-CoV). An outbreak of severe respiratory illness, with high mortality, was first described in Asia in 2002. The epidemic then spread across countries in Asia, North America, South America, and Europe. The last cases were seen in 2004. During the epidemic there were approximately 8,000 cases of severe pneumonia and 800 deaths. Like its fellow corona virus, MERS-CoV, nosocomial spread was seen thus PPE, as for MERS CoV, would be indicated if there was a recurrence.

Non-viral pathogens (such as Histoplasma, Cryptococcus, *Acinetobacter* spp., tuberculosis (TB), *Francisella tularensis*, and *Burkholderia pseudomallei*) in the differential diagnosis are beyond the scope of this chapter.

9.4 What microbiology investigations should be organized?

Rapid diagnostic tests are quick and easy to perform, where resources allow. Virus can be detected in respiratory samples (throat swab, sputum or nasopharyngeal aspirate) using PCR. Typically, a respiratory sample can be tested for a 'panel' of pathogens (multiplex PCR) including respiratory viruses and atypical pathogens including *Mycoplasma pneumoniae, Legionella pneumophila*, and MERS-CoV. During the 'flu season', commercial rapid antigen tests (enzyme immuno-assay (EIA)) on respiratory specimens can give a quick result for influenza and RSV, are less expensive but are less sensitive.

Urinary antigen detection (EIA) tests can be performed for *Legionella pneumophila* (serotype 01 only detected) and *Streptococcus pneumoniae*.

Blood cultures should be performed where sepsis is present along with pneumonia.

A diagnosis of pneumonia (especially in young adults) should prompt testing for **HIV antibody** as pneumonia may be the first presentation of HIV infection and because the spectrum of pathogens differs where advanced HIV infection is present.

9.5 A throat swab is positive for the presence of influenza virus. Does this change your management plan?

Yes. Avian influenza should be strongly considered, especially if the patient has had recent (< 10 days) exposure to either sick or dead birds *or* a human case of avian influenza, *or* if he is a laboratory worker with exposure to avian influenza.

If none of these are the case, then seasonal influenza is the likely diagnosis. Enhanced precautions for MERS-CoV would no longer be needed. Isolation and respiratory precautions should be maintained during the hospital admission of a case of influenza to protect the healthcare worker and other patients.

The mainstay of treatment for influenza infection is supportive management with hydration and symptomatic analgesia. Treatment with anti-influenza agents such as neuraminidase inhibitors (oseltamivir, zanamivir) and less commonly, adamantanes (amantadine, rimantadine) is indicated for immunocompromised patients and certain risk groups including those with chronic respiratory disease (see Case 8). Additionally, exposure of immunocompromised patients to influenza may warrant prophylaxis with neuraminidase inhibitors. National and international guidelines exist for the identification of which patients to treat. Additionally, the prevention of seasonal influenza is important and those at risk should undergo vaccination prior to the onset of the influenza season.

The case described would be a candidate for treatment with an oral influenza treatment, such as oseltamivir (usual dose 75mg twice daily by mouth (bd po) for 5 days) according to UK guidelines as he has a history of asthma.

Further reading

Centers for Disease Control and Prevention, Information on Avian Influenza. https://www.cdc. gov/flu/avianflu/

Public Health England. Avian influenza: guidance, data and analysis. 30 August 2014, updated March 2017. https://www.gov.uk/government/collections/ avian-influenza-guidance-data-and-analysis

Public Health England. MERS-CoV: public health investigation and management of possible cases. July 2014. https://www.gov.uk/government/publications/ mers-cov-public-health-investigation-and-management-of-possible-cases

Public Health England. Middle East Respiratory Syndrome (MERS-CoV) Infection Prevention and Control Guidance. 5 November 2013, updated 20 September 2016. https://www.gov.uk/ government/publications/merscov-infection-control-for-possible-or-confirmed-cases

Case 10

Andrew Woodhouse

Case history

A 45-year-old man presents with a 3-month history of cough, occasional sputum production, intermittent fever, and left-sided chest pain. He has lived in the United Kingdom for 5 years but originates from the Ukraine. His chest X-ray (CXR) shows bilateral infiltrates in the upper zones (Fig. 10.1). Computerized tomography (CT) scan demonstrates cavitating lesions (Fig. 10.2). A sputum sample is direct smear positive for acid-fast bacilli. On further questioning he admits to having been previously treated for tuberculosis (TB) which he acquired during a period of incarceration in a Russian prison 7 years earlier. He is uncertain of the details of his treatment but thinks he completed between 3 and 6 months of treatment consisting of tablets. He doesn't think that he received tablets each day.

Questions

10.1 How much of a concern is drug-resistant TB in a case like this and what initial investigations and management should be instituted?

10.2 What constitutes multi-drug-resistant tuberculosis (MDR-TB) and extensively drug-resistant tuberculosis (XDR-TB)?

10.3 What laboratory testing is available which might give an early indication of drug resistance?

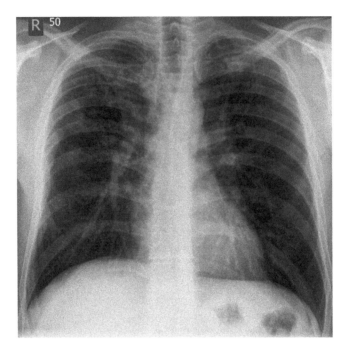

Figure 10.1 Chest X-ray showing bilateral upper zone infiltrates.

Reproduced courtesy of University Hospitals Birmingham NHS Foundation Trust, UK.

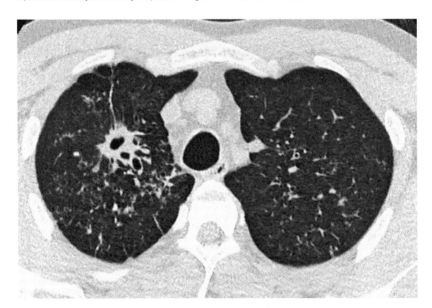

Figure 10.2 High resolution CT thorax showing a cavitating lesion in the right upper lobe with surrounding nodular infiltrate.

Reproduced courtesy of University Hospitals Birmingham NHS Foundation Trust, UK.

Answers

10.1 How much of a concern is drug-resistant TB in a case like this and what initial investigations and management should be instituted?

His history of previous (probably suboptimal) treatment for tuberculosis and acquisition of disease in a setting where high rates of drug-resistant tuberculosis occur are risk factors for drug-resistant disease. He is sputum smear positive and as such represents a significant infectious risk to others. He should be admitted to an isolation facility, preferably a negative pressure isolation room. Further sputum should be sent for microscopy and culture and rapid testing for confirmation of species and preliminary testing for resistance. He needs baseline blood tests including testing for HIV infection, something which should be offered to all patients with tuberculosis. In this case, testing for other blood borne viruses is indicated due to a high risk of hepatitis C infection in prison.

10.2 What constitutes multi-drug-resistant tuberculosis (MDR-TB) and extensively drug-resistant tuberculosis (XDR-TB)?

Multi-drug-resistant tuberculosis is defined by resistance to both isoniazid and rifampicin, the two most effective first line anti-tuberculous drugs. Resistance to one or other drug plus resistance to other first-line agents (streptomycin, pyrazinamide, and ethambutol) does not meet the definition of MDR-TB but still represents an important treatment challenge. Mono drug resistance to isoniazid is the commonest form of tuberculosis resistance seen worldwide but rates of MDR-TB are rising.

Extensively drug resistant tuberculosis is MDR-TB plus resistance to at least one fluoroquinolone *and* to one of the injectable agents (amikacin, kanamycin, capreomycin). While overall numbers remain low, XDR-TB has been diagnosed across the world with over 100 countries reporting cases. The highest numbers of XDR-TB cases as a proportion of MDR-TB are in countries from the former Soviet Union. The highest absolute numbers of XDR-TB cases are in China, India, South Africa, and the Philippines.

10.3 What laboratory testing is available which might give an early indication of drug resistance?

The gold standard for identifying drug resistance in TB at present depends on drug susceptibility testing (DST). This takes considerable time (weeks to months) as it requires culture of the organism and then phenotypic resistance testing. More recently, rapid, technically straightforward molecular tests have been approved and are widely available which can provide useful early information.

The Xpert MTB/RIF (Cepheid) test is a PCR assay used directly on diagnostic samples. Test material, usually sputum, is directly transferred into a cartridge after minor preparation steps. The process is then fully automated. The result is confirmation of *M. tuberculosis* complex and detection of the major mutations in the *rpoB* gene which account for 98% of resistance to rifampicin. This result can be available within hours of the laboratory receiving the sample. Identification of rifampicin resistance implies a high likelihood of at least MDR-TB and appropriate infection control precautions and contact tracing can be undertaken. The GenoType MTBDR*plus* (Hain-Lifescience) is a line probe assay that can detect resistance to both isoniazid and rifampicin and has been endorsed by the World Health Organization (WHO) for use on respiratory samples and on organisms from positive cultures from other sites. There are additional preparation steps compared to the MTB/RIF test but results can be available within 5–6 hours. The GenoType MTBDR*sl* has been developed which can detect resistance to quinolones and aminoglycosides, thereby allowing early identification of XDR-TB. An emerging technology currently under clinical evaluation is whole genome sequencing (WGS) which can be performed once an organism is growing in culture. WGS of a TB culture will potentially revolutionize identification and treatment of resistant TB by identifying predictive susceptibility profiles for most of the available treatment drugs. Results from WGS are available well before phenotypic susceptibility tests can be completed.

Case history continued

The day after admission the laboratory calls to say that PCR and line probe assay have confirmed *M. tuberculosis* with genotypic features suggesting resistance to both isoniazid and rifampicin.

Questions

10.4 What drug treatment options are available in this situation?

10.5 What would be reasonable drug treatment to commence while awaiting extended sensitivities?

10.6 What drug toxicity issues are important in the treatment of MDR- and XDR-TB?

10.7 What are the outcomes of treatment of MDR- and XDR-TB?

Answers

10.4 What drug treatment options are available in this situation?

He has at least MDR-TB based on the genetic tests and therefore any treatment schedule must be appropriate for MDR-TB. There remains a possibility of XDR-TB but further susceptibility information will take longer to be reported. Treatment protocols for MDR-TB are evolving and the WHO has produced recommendations to guide treatment and to try to introduce a consistent approach globally. These recommendations were revised in 2018. The most recent WHO recommendations for the treatment of MDR-TB are shown in Table 10.1. Importantly there is reduced emphasis on including injectable agents and in particular, capreomycin and kanamycin are no longer recommended for use.

10.5 What would be reasonable drug treatment to commence while awaiting extended sensitivities?

A core initial MDR-TB treatment regimen should include 5 drugs. It is recommended that the combination includes a quinolone plus bedaquiline and linezolid (Group A)

Table 10.1 Drug groups for treatment of MDR-TB

WHO Drug group	Antibiotic	Comment
Group A. Include all three medicines	Levofloxacin or moxifloxacin	Unless cannot be used for other reasons
	Bedaquiline	
	Linezolid	
Group B. Add both medicines	Clofazimine	Unless cannot be used for other reasons
	Cycloserine or terizidone	
Group C. Add to complete the regimen and when drugs from Groups A and B cannot be used.	Ethambutol	
	Delamanid	
	Pyrazinamide	
	Imipenem-cilastatin or meropenem	Amoxicillin-clavulanate used alongside for clavulanate component
	Amikacin or streptomycin	Injectable agents
	Ethionamide or prothionamide	
	Para-aminosalycilic acid (PAS)	

Adapted with permission from World Health Organization (WHO). (2018). *Rapid communication: Key changes to treatment of multidrug- and rifampicin-resistant tuberculosis (MDR/RR-TB)*.http://www.who.int/tb/publications/2018/WHO_RapidCommunicationMDRTB.pdf.

to which is added clofazamine and cycloserine/terizidone (Group B drugs). If any of these drugs are unable to be used then drugs from group C should be added, working from the order they appear on the list in Table 10.1.

- Treatment of MDR- and XDR-TB is complex and requires careful monitoring due to the potential for drug toxicity. Treatment should be under the supervision of or in close communication with a clinician experienced in the management of such cases.

10.6 What drug toxicity issues are important in the treatment of MDR- and XDR-TB?

While all drugs have potential adverse effects there are particular issues with some of the drugs used in the treatment of MDR- and XDR-TB.

A number of the agents can cause QT interval prolongation including the fluoroquinolones, bedaquiline, delaminid, and clofazamine. Electrocardiogram

Table 10.2 Resistant TB treatment side effects and monitoring

Antibiotic	Selected adverse effects	Monitoring/comments
Fluoroquinolones	Tendinopathy QT interval prolongation	Clinical ECG monitoring: baseline, 2 weeks, 1–3 monthly.
Aminoglycosides	Nephrotoxicity Ototoxicity Vestibular dysfunction	Renal function Audiometry: baseline, 2 weeks then monthly.
Ethionamide/ protionamide	Hypothyroidism	Thyroid function tests (TFTs)
Cycloserine	Neurologic: confusion, somnolence, depression, suicidal ideation.	Clinical
Linezolid	Myelosuppression	Regular FBC
Clofazamine	Skin discolouration QT prolongation	Warn patients ECG monitoring: baseline, 2 weeks, 1–3 monthly.
PAS	Hypothyroidism (more likely if concomitant protionamide)	TFTs.
Bedaquiline	Arthralgia, chest pain, nausea, headache, haemoptysis QT prolongation	Clinical ECG monitoring: baseline, 2 weeks, monthly.
Delaminid	Dermatitis, urticaria, nausea, dizziness, haemoptysis QT prolongation	Clinical ECG monitoring: baseline, 2 weeks, monthly.

PAS, para-amino salicyclic; Source: data from TB Drug Monographs, http://www.tbdrugmonographs.co.uk/.

(ECG) monitoring is required in patients on these drugs. Linezolid may cause myelosuppression.

Aminoglycosides, if required, are used for prolonged periods, usually at least 3–6 months. Patients should be monitored for nephrotoxicity, ototoxicity, and vestibular dysfunction. Baseline audiometry should be performed followed by at least monthly examinations.

Protionamide and *p*-aminosalicylic acid (PAS) may both cause hypothyroidism, with a greater risk if used in combination.

Table 10.2 is a summary of some important potential adverse effects which may arise during treatment of drug-resistant TB. Detailed information should be obtained from product monographs.

10.7 What are the outcomes of treatment of MDR- and XDR-TB?

The outcome of treatment of MDR- and XDR-TB varies from country to country but is challenging even in high-resource healthcare environments. The WHO collates outcome data from regions across the globe and the most recent published outcome data indicates cure rates of around 60% for MDR-TB and 30% for XDR-TB.

Further reading

Boehme CC, Nabeta P, Hillesmanne D, Nichol MP, Shenai S, et al. Rapid molecular detection of tuberculosis and rifampicin resistance. *N Engl J Med* 2010; **363**:1005–15.

Dheda K, Barry CE, Maartens G. Tuberculosis. *Lancet* 2016; **387**: 1211–26.

Ghandhi NR, Nunn P, Dheda K, Schaaf HS, Zignol M, et al. Multidrug-resistant and extensively drug resistant tuberculosis: a threat to global control of tuberculosis. *Lancet* 2010; **375**:1830–43.

Global tuberculosis report 2017. Geneva: World Health Organization; 2017. Licence: CC BY-NCSA 3.0 IGO.

World Health Organization. 2019. WHO consolidated guidelines on drug-resistant tuberculosis treatment. License CC BY-NC-SA. 3.0 IGO.

Case 11

Andrew Woodhouse

Case history

A 42-year-old man presents with a cough that has been present for 18 days following an initial 1-week illness consisting of nasal congestion, sneezing, and conjunctival injection. He has been referred to the hospital ambulatory medical clinic for review, and a chest X-ray (CXR). He is a non-smoker, his CXR is normal, and a full blood count shows a lymphocytosis. He was born in the United Kingdom and so far as he is aware received all vaccinations recommended during childhood and adolescence. Your differential diagnosis includes whooping cough because of the duration of the cough.

The patient has two children aged 6 and 8 years and his partner is 36 weeks pregnant. The children have been immunized according to recommended schedules. His partner has not had any vaccinations since childhood.

Questions

11.1 How would you confirm a diagnosis of *Bordetella pertussis* infection?

11.2 What antibiotic treatment, if any, is indicated for the patient?

11.3 What should be advised regarding antibiotic 'prophylaxis' for the family?

11.4 What is the role of post-exposure pertussis vaccination of contacts and should any of the family contacts be offered vaccination?

11.5 What non-antibiotic treatment options might be considered for someone with persistent, protracted cough due to pertussis?

Answers

11.1 How would you confirm a diagnosis of *Bordetella pertussis* infection?

A presumptive diagnosis of whooping cough can be made using a clinical case definition such as a cough lasting 14 days or more with one characteristic symptom—a 'whoop', post-cough vomiting, or paroxysms of cough. These classical symptoms are less likely to be seen in patients who have been immunized previously. Confirmation of infection is made by culture of *B. pertussis* from a nasopharyngeal aspirate or per nasal swab. Culture is most likely to be positive during the first two weeks of illness. PCR can also detect evidence of infection and is likely to be positive for longer. Ideally both culture and PCR should be sent from patients with symptoms for less than 3 weeks. Beyond 3 weeks the yield falls, especially from culture, although the combination of the two tests will result in higher detection rates than either alone. The positive yield of both tests is less in previously immunized people.

Serology to detect IgG (immunoglobulin G) antibodies to pertussis toxin can be used and is helpful in adolescent and adult patients with cough lasting over 2 weeks, provided they have not received pertussis immunization within the last year. In the United Kingdom, an anti-pertussis toxin antibody level of greater than 70 IU/ml is considered serological evidence of infection in such cases.

11.2 What antibiotic treatment, if any, is indicated for the patient?

Antibiotic treatment has limited impact on the clinical illness but it does reduce transmission of the organism and eradicates carriage, hence it is used as a public health measure to reduce the number of secondary cases. Macrolides are recommended, historically erythromycin, but more recently clarithromycin and azithromycin have become the drugs of choice. Co-trimoxazole is an alternative for those with a macrolide intolerance. Treatment should be given as early as possible for maximum benefit and should be started if whooping cough is suspected. After 21 days of illness, patients are no longer infectious and antibiotics are not indicated. If treatment is indicated a 5-day course of azithromycin or 7 days of clarithromycin or erythromycin are recommended compared to 14 days of co-trimoxazole.

11.3 What should be advised regarding antibiotic 'prophylaxis' for the family?

There is limited evidence for the benefit of antibiotic prophylaxis of close and household contacts. Nonetheless recommendations exist which stratify advice depending on risk group. Individuals who are considered 'vulnerable' are those at increased risk of developing severe complications following pertussis infection—essentially, unimmunized infants and children. Those at risk of transmitting infection (i.e. symptomatic patients) to such vulnerable individuals if they themselves were to develop pertussis are also considered in prophylaxis decisions. In the United Kingdom, for example, antibiotic prophylaxis is recommended for close household contacts of a case within 21 days of onset of symptoms in either the vulnerable or at risk of transmission groups.

In the United Kingdom, the children would be considered fully immunized and would have received pertussis vaccine at 2, 3, and 4 months with a pre-school booster. They would not routinely be offered antibiotic prophylaxis.

The pregnant woman falls into the transmission risk group because she is over 32-weeks gestation and has not received the vaccine within the last 5 years. The concern is potential transmission to her newborn baby should she develop pertussis infection and be unwell during the delivery period. Neonates are at risk of serious complications of pertussis including death, hence the importance of preventing transmission. Erythromycin is the recommended antibiotic in pregnancy.

11.4 What is the role of post-exposure pertussis vaccination of contacts and should any of the family contacts be offered vaccination?

The duration of protection from immunization with pertussis vaccine is not precisely known but is not lifelong and is likely to be less than 10 years. Unimmunized or partially immunized children under 10 years should receive post-exposure vaccination. The UK advice has extended this to household contacts over 10 years of age who are at risk of transmitting pertussis to vulnerable individuals if the contacts, exposed to pertussis, have not been vaccinated in the last 5 years. This includes pregnant women of 32+ weeks gestation, healthcare workers caring for infants and pregnant women, other workers with close contact with young children who have not been fully vaccinated, and household contacts of very young, incompletely immunized children.

In the scenario outlined in Question 11.3, the patient's pregnant partner is a candidate for post-exposure vaccination in addition to antibiotic prophylaxis. In the United Kingdom, the United States, Ireland, Australia, and New Zealand it is recommended that pregnant women receive a booster dose of vaccine during their pregnancy. Vaccination during pregnancy not only protects a mother exposed to pertussis but there is also passive protection of the newborn infant through transplacental transfer of maternal antibody.

11.5 What non-antibiotic treatment options might be considered for someone with persistent, protracted cough due to pertussis?

A variety of cough treatments have been proposed for whooping cough including corticosteroids, β-adrenergic agonists, antihistamines, and pertussis-specific immunoglobulin. A systematic review of the subject found a poor-quality evidence base for their efficacy and no conclusions could be drawn as to the effectiveness of various interventions for cough.

Further reading

Guidelines for the Public Health Management of Pertussis in England. Public Health England. July 2016. Available at: https://www.gov.uk/government/publications/pertussis-guidelines-for-public-health-management.

Gopal DP, Barber J, Toeg D. Pertussis (Whooping cough) *Br Med J* 2019; **364**: 1401. doi:10.1136/bmj.1401.

Guiso N, Berbers G, Fry NK , He Q, Gissman S, et al. What to do and what not to do in serological diagnosis of pertussis: recommendations from EU reference laboratories. *Eur J Clin Microbiol Infect Dis* 2011; **30**: 307–12.

Kilgore P, Salim AM, Zervos MJ, Schmitt HJ. Pertussis: microbiology, disease, treatment, and prevention. *Clin Microbiol Rev* 2016; **3**: 449–86.

Wang K, Bettiol S, Thompson MJ, Roberts NW, Perera R, et al. Symptomatic treatment of the cough in whooping cough. *Cochrane Database of Systematic Reviews* 2014, Issue 9, Art.no. CD003257. doi:10.1002/14651858.CD003257.pub5.

Case 12

Bridget L. Atkins

Case history

A 45-year-old teacher has completed induction therapy for acute myeloid leukaemia. She presents with a 3-day history of cough and pleuritic chest pain. She is mildly short of breath on exertion. On examination she is alert and fully orientated. Her temperature is 38.3 °C. Oxygen saturation is 94% on room air. Respiratory rate is 16. Blood pressure is normal, and the heart rate is 96 beats per minute (bpm). She has reduced breath sounds bilaterally and some scattered crepitations. The rest of her physical examination is unremarkable. Her chest X-ray (CXR) is normal. Bloods show neutropenia ($< 0.1 \times 10^9$/L).

Questions

12.1   What further investigations would you perform on day 1?

12.2   What treatment would you give her initially?

Answers

12.1 What further investigations would you perform on day 1?

The presence of fever and respiratory symptoms and signs in a neutropaenic patient means that a lower respiratory infection is likely. Blood cultures should be taken; sputum or induced sputum should be obtained if possible and a viral throat swab should be sent for respiratory viruses. A high-resolution computerized tomography (CT) scan of the chest should be performed promptly.

12.2 What treatment would you give her initially?

Empirically, a broad spectrum β-lactam antibiotic with activity against pseudomonas should be initiated in line with local guidelines for neutropenic sepsis. Neuraminidase inhibitors should be considered during influenza season. In addition, an aminoglycoside should be considered if the patient is haemodynamically compromised or at risk of multi-drug resistant (MDR) Gram-negative sepsis. The duration of aminoglycoside should be reviewed within 48 hours because of the risk of oto- and nephrotoxicity.

Case history continued

A CT scan of the chest is performed. This shows several areas of patchy consolidation bilaterally, nodules and a halo sign.

Questions

12.3 What is the differential diagnosis of these clinical and radiological findings?

12.4 What other radiological features could you look for?

12.5 Describe the epidemiology of fungal infections in haematology patients

12.6 What further laboratory investigations should be considered?

12.7 How would you modify treatment?

Answers

12.3 What is the differential diagnosis of these clinical and radiological findings?

Lung infiltrates in the immunocompromised host can arise from infective or non-infective causes. Non-infective causes include drug toxicity, leukaemic infiltration, pulmonary oedema, and/or haemorrhage. Infective causes include viruses, bacteria, yeasts and filamentous fungi, and *Pneumocystis jirovecii* pneumonia.

Common upper respiratory viruses can progress to lower respiratory tract infection (LRTI) in compromised patients (e.g. influenza, RSV, para-influenza, human metapneumovirus, and adenoviruses). Other upper respiratory viruses (e.g. rhinovirus, corona viruses, bocavirus, polyoma viruses) appear less likely to cause LRTI. Cytomegalovirus can also cause pneumonia in the immunocompromised although this is more of a significant problem in those who have received an allogeneic haematopoietic stem cell transplant (HSCT).

Bacterial lung infections may include classical pathogens such as *Streptococcus pneumoniae* or less commonly with 'atypical' pneumonia agents (*Legionella*,- *Mycoplasma*, and *Chlamydophila* spp.). A range of (sometimes MDR) Gram-positive and Gram-negative bacteria could cause lung infection in these hosts. *Stenotrophomonas maltophilia* is being increasingly reported as a cause of life-threatening haemorrhagic pneumonia in some parts of the world.

Pneumocystis jirovecii infections are increasingly being reported in immune-compromised patients but the classical CT appearance is with central diffuse ground-glass infiltrates with sparing of the periphery.

Nocardia spp. should be considered in patients with solid organ transplantation, steroid therapy, alcoholism, diabetes, and/or chronic obstructive pulmonary disease (COPD). This can present with lobar or multilobar consolidation but there are commonly solitary lung masses and/or large nodules. Mycobacterial infections should also be considered in specific risk groups such as HIV-infected patients or those on disease-modifying monoclonal antibodies such as infliximab.

In this case with severe neutropaenia and consolidation with macronodules (> 1 cm), an invasive filamentous fungal infection, most likely *Aspergillus* spp. is likely. Other filamentous fungi such as the Zygomycetes and *Scedesporium* spp. should be considered but are less common.

12.4 What other radiological features could you look for?

Radiological features that support the diagnosis of invasive aspergillosis include nodules (which can also occur in viral infections), a halo sign (a nodule surrounded by a ground-glass halo), and an air crescent sign (a crescentic collection of air separating a nodule or mass from the wall of a surrounding cavity) (Fig. 12.1) (Fig. 12.2). The latter two are suggestive of angioinvasive aspergillus infection. A reverse

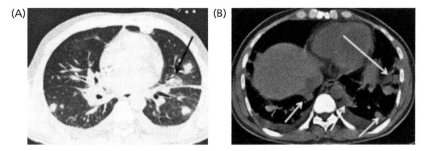

Figure 12.1 (A) Computed tomography (CT) images obtained in a 45-year-old man with angio-invasive pulmonary aspergillosis and who had received a hematopoietic stem cell transplant 13 months previously. (A) High resolution CT lung image (1-mm thick) obtained at the level of the lower pulmonary veins. Image shows ill-defined macronodules with halo signs in both lungs. Note the nodule with an air-crescent sign in the left upper lobe (arrow). (B) Conventional CT mediastinal image (5-mm thick) obtained at the level of the right hemidiaphragm. The image shows bilateral pleural effusion. Note the wedge-shaped consolidations (short arrows) in both lower lobes, and the internal cavities in the lateral basal segment of the left lower lobe (long arrow), which indicates lung infarctions by angioinvasion.

Reproduced with permission from Kim S, et al. (2015). Invasive Pulmonary Aspergillosis-mimicking Tuberculosis. *Clin Infect Dis*. 61(1):9–17. Copyright © 2015, Oxford University Press. DOI: https://doi.org/10.1093/cid/civ216.

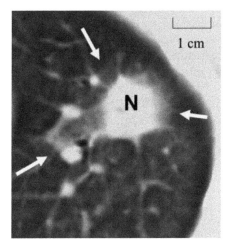

Figure 12.2 Computed tomographic section through the lung, demonstrating a halo sign. The sign consists of 2 parts: a solid nodular core (N), through which no pulmonary parenchyma is visible, and a ground-glass perimeter of intermediate density (arrows) through which pulmonary parenchyma is still visible. Note that the nodule is > 1 cm in diameter and that the area of ground-glass opacity surrounds more than three-quarters of the nodule.

Reproduced with permission from Green RG, et al. (2007). Imaging Findings in Acute Invasive Pulmonary Aspergillosis: Clinical Significance of the Halo Sign. *Clin Infect Dis*. 44(3):373–379. DOI: https://doi.org/10.1086/509917.

halo sign (or reverse birds nest sign) consists of irregular intersecting areas of stranding or irregular lines within areas of ground-glass opacity and is more suggestive of mucormycosis.

12.5 Describe the epidemiology of fungal infections in immunocompromised patients

Aspergillus spp., Zygomycetes (including Mucor), and other moulds are ubiquitous saprophytes present in air, soil, and water; therefore, exposure to these agents is almost universal. The primary mode of acquiring these infections is inhalation of fungal spores. After inhalation, spores are deposited in the mucous membranes of the upper and lower respiratory tract, and this may lead to pulmonary or sinus infection in extremely susceptible immunocompromised patients.

Patients at greatest risk for invasive fungal disease are those with acute myeloid leukaemia (including in first induction), allogeneic HSCT (particularly with cord blood source), and heart, lung, or liver transplantation.

12.6 What further laboratory investigations can be considered?

Further investigations should include a bronchoscopy and washings if the patient can tolerate this. A multiplex PCR for respiratory virus can be performed on this (or on upper respiratory samples if lower samples not possible). Cultures should be performed for bacteria and fungi. Immunofluoresence and PCR should be performed for *Pneumocystis jirovecii* but there is no reliable cut-off for PCR to differentiate colonization from infection.

Biomarkers (such as galactomannan and β-D glucan) on serum and broncho-alveolar lavage (BAL) samples for diagnostic purposes have a role but lack good specificity and sensitivity. Aspergillus PCR and/or a lateral flow (monoclonal antibody) test for *Aspergillus* spp. can be performed on respiratory samples. However, a negative result in this patient is unlikely to affect the decision to treat. Biomarkers and aspergillus PCR may have a role in the pre-emptive screening of high-risk patients prior to developing symptoms.

12.7 How would you modify treatment?

Voriconazole is the primary antifungal of choice in this patient with suspected aspergillus. Alternatives include lipid formulations of amphotericin B, echinocandins such as caspofungin or micafungin, or newer azoles such as posaconazole or isavuconazole. Combination treatment has not been shown to be superior to monotherapy but may be considered for salvage therapy. Some species of aspergillus (e.g. *Aspergillus terreus*) have reduced susceptibility to amphotericin B so full identification of the fungus is essential. Azole resistance in *Aspergillus fumigatus* has now been reported in several countries and may be responsible for treatment failures.

Further reading

Chemaly RF, Shah DP, Boeckh MJ. Management of respiratory viral infections in hematopoietic cell transplant recipients and patients with hematologic malignancies. *Clin Infect Dis* 2014; **59**: S344–51.

Greene RE, Schlamm HT, Oestmann JW, Stark P, Durand C, et al. Imaging findings in acute invasive pulmonary aspergillosis: clinical significance of the halo sign. *Clin Infect Dis* 2007; **44**: 373–9.

Robert-Gangneux F, Belaz S, Revest M, Tattevin P, Jouneau S, et al. Diagnosis of *Pneumocystis jirovecii* pneumonia in immunocompromised patients by real-time PCR: a 4-year prospective study. *J Clin Microbiol* 2014; **52**: 3370–6.

Patterson TF, Thompson III GR, Denning DW, Fishman JA, Hadley S, et al. Practice guidelines for the diagnosis and management of aspergillosis: 2016 update by the Infectious Diseases Society of America. *Clin Infect Dis* 2016; **63**: e1–e60.

Ullmann AJ, Aguado JM, Arikan-Akdagli S, Denning DW, Groll AH, et al. Diagnosis and management of Aspergillus diseases: executive summary of the 2017 ESCMID-ECMM-ERS guideline. *Clin Microbiol Infect* 2018; **24**: e1–e38.

Case 13

Hilary Humphreys

Case history

A 23-year-old male patient presents to Cystic Fibrosis Outpatients with a productive cough and purulent sputum. He has noticed increased breathlessness on moderate exertion compared to previously, and today's pulmonary function tests show some deterioration, compared to the last visit. He is known to be colonized with *Pseudomonas aeruginosa* and *Staphylococcus aureus* and was recently treated with antimicrobial agents targeted against these bacteria. The most recent sputum grew *Stenotrophomonas maltophilia*.

Questions

13.1 What is *Stenotrophomonas maltophilia* and what is its likely significance in this patient?

13.2 What laboratory methods should be used for the recovery and identification of *S. maltophilia*?

Answers

13.1 What is *Stenotrophomonas maltophilia* and what is its likely significance in this patient?

S. maltophilia was originally classified as a pseudomonas and is an environmental bacterium found in the soil. It is increasingly recognized as an opportunist pathogen in immunocompromised patients such as those with malignancy, in intensive care units, and in patients with cystic fibrosis (CF). Risk factors in CF patients include increasing age and recent oral antibiotics. In patients with CF, it may cause transient colonization, persistent infection or occasionally acute exacerbations. There is no convincing evidence to date that it is readily transmitted from person to person. Other non-fermentative environmental Gram-negative bacilli are increasingly isolated from CF patients. However, decisions on whether to treat will depend on the clinical condition of the patient. In this patient, it may be responsible for the deterioration in lung function.

13.2 What laboratory methods should be used for the recovery and identification of *S. maltophilia*?

The processing of respiratory specimens from patients with CF is increasingly challenging and requires considerable laboratory expertise. In addition to processing for *P. aeruginosa*, *Haemophilus influenzae*, and *S. aureus*, often the initial causes of exacerbations, it is necessary to culture for *Burkholderia* spp., *Aspergillus* spp., nontuberculous mycobacteria, and fungi (e.g. *Aspergillus* spp.) which have emerged in older patients as the life expectancy of the CF cohort increases.

All non-fermenting Gram-negative bacilli should be identified to species level and Gram-negative selective agar has been recommended for routine use to detect their presence, in addition to selective media for *Burkholderia cepacia* complex. One such selective medium for Gram-negative bacilli incorporates vancomycin, amphotericin B, and imipenem. Recent treatment with carbapenem antibiotics predisposes to colonization and infection with *S. maltophilia* which is intrinsically resistant to these agents. This explains the use of imipenem in selective media for its recovery from sputum.

Currently, there are no recognized and validated molecular methods for the identification of *S. maltophilia*. Increasingly, matrix-assisted laser desorption/ionization time-of-flight mass spectrometry (MALDI-TOF) mass spectrometry is used as a phenotypic method of identification. This system of mass spectrometry allows for the analysis of large organic molecules, which includes three stages: mixing of sample with matrix material, laser irradiation triggering ablation and desorption, and then ionization. From a colony on an agar plate, MALDI-TOF can identify a broad range of bacteria and fungi in minutes and has significantly improved turnaround times in the diagnostic laboratory.

Case history continued

The patient is admitted with a view to a full assessment of his current status. After review and discussion with the patient, specific intravenous antibiotics for *S. maltophilia* are commenced in addition to the continuation of his inhaled antibiotics. However, the in-patient CF unit has a high bed occupancy rate and not every bed is in a single room. Discussions take place regarding where he might be best placed.

Questions

13.3 What are the treatment considerations in this patient?

13.4 What is the role of inhaled antibiotics in patients with CF?

13.5 Should this patient be isolated?

13.6 What other infection prevention and control measures are indicated in hospitals?

Answers

13.3 What are the treatment considerations in this patient?

The culture result may represent colonization or be the cause of or be contributing to his symptoms and deteriorating lung function. Given recent treatment for combined staphylococcal and pseudomonal infection, it can be difficult to determine the clinical significance of the most recent sputum culture result. *S. maltophilia* is resistant to many commonly used antibiotics and consequently susceptibility testing should be carried out against trimethoprim-sulfamethoxazole, doxycycline, and chloramphenicol, amongst others. If susceptible, co-trimoxazole is the treatment of choice. Table 13.1 outlines some features of opportunist Gram-negative pathogens in CF and possible options for treatment.

13.4 What is the role of inhaled antibiotics in patients with CF?

Evidence suggests that inhaled antibiotics are cost-effective and reduce pulmonary exacerbations. The most commonly used inhaled antibiotics are colistin and tobramycin, and both are recommended as eradication therapy in early *P. aeruginosa* infection. Other agents that can be administered by this route include aztreonam, levofloxacin, and liposomal amikacin. Given the differing pharmacokinetics of antibiotics in patients with CF and the possibility of achieving high concentrations at the site of infection, inhaled antibiotics are an attractive alternative to intravenous

Table 13.1 Emerging opportunist Gram-negative bacilli in patients with cystic fibrosis other than *Burkholderia* spp.

Pathogen	Natural habitat	Role in CF	Treatment
Stenotrophomonas maltophilia	Soil, hospital sinks, faucets	Transient or recurrent infection	Co-trimoxazole is the drug of choice
Achromobacter alcaligenes (xylosoxidans)	Water, fluids in hospitals including decolonized water	Isolated from 2–30% of patients; varies with population and laboratory methodology	Guided by susceptibility testing with some caveats
Ralstonia spp.	Soil, rivers, lakes, contaminated solutions	Asymptomatic colonization and pneumonia	May be multi antibiotic resistance but *in-vitro* testing may not reflect *in-vivo* activity

antibiotics, either for treatment, or for the long-term suppression of pseudomonas colonization.

13.5 Should this patient be isolated?

Yes. Many recent guidelines strongly recommend the admission of all patients with CF, regardless of known or unknown bacterial colonization/infection, to an individual single room when hospitalization is required, preferably in a designated CF unit. This is mainly to reduce the transmission of multi-drug-resistant *P. aeruginosa* and *B. cepacia* during coughing to other patients and to optimize patient care. Single rooms for patients with CF should have controlled ventilation to diminish the risk of airborne spread (Fig. 13.1). In the absence of ventilation, rooms should be left vacant for between 30 minutes and 1 hour to allow settlement of all airborne particles before cleaning.

13.6 What other infection prevention and control measures are indicated in hospitals?

In the United States, healthcare workers are advised to use gloves and long-sleeve gowns for all occasions including mere contact with the patient's surroundings, and patients should also wear surgical masks. In Europe, long-sleeve gowns are

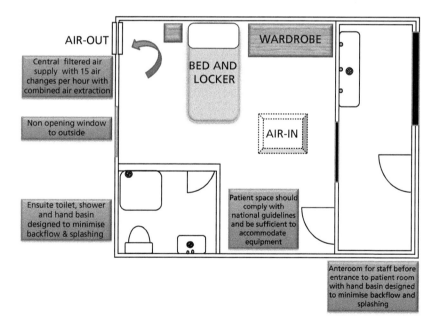

Figure 13.1 Suggested layout of single room for patient with cystic fibrosis.

recommended for physical contact with patients only and surgical masks may be worn by patients when in common ward areas or by healthcare workers as part of droplet precautions.

Acknowledgements

Acknowledgement to Niall Stevens, Anna-Rose Prior, and Margaret Gillham

Further reading

Chang Y-T, Lin C-Y, Chen Y-H, Hsueh P-R. Update on infections caused by *Stenotrophomonas maltophilia* with particular attention to resistance mechanisms and therapeutic options. *Front Microbiol* 2015; **6**: 893. doi: 10.3389/fmicb.2015.00893.

Döring G, Flume P, Heijerman H, Elborn JS. Treatment of lung infection in patients with cystic fibrosis: Current and future strategies. *J Cystic Fibrosis* 2012; **11**: 461–79.

Schaffer K. Epidemiology of infection and current guidelines for infection prevention in cystic fibrosis patients. *J Hosp Infect* 2015; **89**: 309–13.

The UK Cystic Fibrosis Trust Microbiology Laboratory Standards Working Group. Laboratory standards for processing microbiological samples from people with cystic fibrosis. September 2010.

Waters V, Smyth A. Cystic fibrosis microbiology: advances in antimicrobial therapy. *J Cystic Fibrosis* 2015; **14**: 551–60.

Case 14

Hilary Humphreys

Case history

A 55-year-old male presents to hospital with a low-grade pyrexia, non-productive cough, and increasing dyspnoea. Nine months previously, he had a cadaveric kidney transplant and he is currently on maintenance immunosuppressive therapy of tacrolimus, mycophenolate sodium, and prednisone. His initial investigations, including a full blood count, urea and electrolytes, and liver function tests, are all normal. His chest X-ray (CXR) shows diffuse interstitial infiltrates in the left mid zone. Urine for pneumococcal and legionella antigens is taken as are nasopharyngeal swabs for a possible viral cause, and blood cultures. He is commenced on intravenous pipercillin-tazobactam and clarithromycin. However, he does not improve, the results of the microbiological investigations already taken are negative, and 48 hours later he requires intubation and ventilation. Vancomycin and caspofungin are added to his empiric antimicrobial treatment regimen, but despite this, he remains critically ill. A computerized tomography (CT) scan of the thorax shows multiple pulmonary nodules and a nodules and a broncho-alveolar lavage (BAL) is undertaken. Yeast-like organisms are seen on Gram stain of the BAL.

Questions

14.1 Does the presence of yeast-like organisms in the BAL confirm a diagnosis of candida pneumonia?

14.2 What are the clinical characteristics of the likely infection here, and how is it usually diagnosed?

14.3 What is the epidemiology of the pathogen involved?

Answers

14.1 Does the presence of yeast-like organisms in the BAL confirm a diagnosis of pneumonia caused by yeasts?

No. *Candida albicans* or other yeasts in BAL specimens usually represents colonization. Routine microscopy and culture cannot be used to confirm a diagnosis of fungal pneumonia, even for aspergillus infection in an at-risk patient. A diagnosis of infection with *Cryptococcus neoformans*, a true yeast and a likely cause here, even if seen on microscopy, would require histological confirmation in tissue or by some other method as discussed below.

14.2 What are the clinical characteristics of the likely infection here, and how is it usually diagnosed?

The symptoms of cryptococcal infection are often non-specific, as in the case described here, and a high index of clinical suspicion is required in patients with recognized risk factors which include HIV/AIDS, solid organ transplantation, end-stage liver disease, haematological malignancy, patients on anti-TNF-α (anti-tumour necrosis factor alpha) therapy, and steroid-dependent sarcoidosis. Blood, cerebrospinal fluid (CSF), and BAL for cryptococcal antigen testing and culture are used to make a diagnosis and antigen titres usually decline with treatment. Tissue specimens should be subjected to specialized stains such as Gomori methenamine, silver, or periodic acid-Schiff.

14.3 What is the epidemiology of the pathogen involved?

Cryptococcus is ubiquitous and has an extensive habitat in nature. Typically, *C. neoformans* is associated with bird droppings and nests and with infection in temperate climates. *C. gattii* is increasingly recognized but is more commonly found in warmer climates and has been associated with eucalyptus trees. In the 1990s, this species emerged as a significant cause of disease in north-western parts of the United States and British Columbia.

Case history continued

Cryptococcal antigen is positive in the patient's blood and BAL specimens and yeasts are seen on histological staining of tissue taken at BAL, all of which confirm the diagnosis of systemic cryptococcosis with pulmonary involvement. The patient is started on liposomal amphotericin B.

Questions

14.4 What other investigations should be done in this patient, either before or at the time of initiating the anti-cryptococcal treatment?

14.5 What are the other manifestations of cryptococcal disease?

14.6 Why did the patient not respond to the addition of caspofungin when transferred to the intensive care unit (ICU)?

14.7 What is the standard treatment for cryptococcosis?

14.8 Is it possible that this patient acquired the cryptococcal infection from the transplanted kidney?

Answers

14.4 What other investigations should be done in this patient, either before or at the time of initiating the anti-cryptococcal treatment?

This patient should have a lumbar puncture to determine whether there is central nervous system involvement, that is, meningo-encephalitis. The presence of cryptococcus in the central nervous system (CNS) such as seen on microscopy (Fig. 14.1), or via India ink stain on CSF (less commonly used now), culture, or through latex antigen detection, confirms the diagnosis and influences the management strategy as discussed below. Latex agglutination is very reliable with a false positive rate of less than 1%, and high titres (e.g. > 1:1024) suggests a high yeast burden with a greater risk of death. The development of antigen detection through lateral flow assays is significant for income poor settings as there are minimal laboratory requirements and this can be performed as a point-of-care assay.

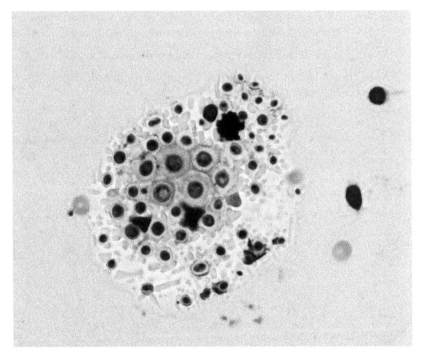

Figure 14.1 May–Grunwald stain of a cytospin preparation of a CSF sample showing yeasts subsequently identified as *C. neoformans* (see colour plate).

Reproduced courtesy of Michael Farrell, Beaumont Hospital, Dublin, Ireland.

14.5 What are the other manifestations of cryptococcal disease?

Apart from infection of the lungs and central nervous system, cryptococcal infection can involve the skin (e.g. nodules and papules), eyes resulting in sight loss, and less occasionally, the urogenital tract and bone.

14.6 Why did the patient not respond to the addition of caspofungin when transferred to the ICU?

The echinocandins have little activity against cryptococcus. Amphotericin B, flucytosine, and the azoles, especially fluconazole, are the mainstays of therapy.

14.7 What is the standard treatment for cryptococcosis?

This largely depends on whether the patient has underlying immune-suppression, and the location and severity of the infection. Recent guidelines emphasize the need for initial induction therapy administered for a matter of weeks followed by consolidation therapy with subsequent maintenance therapy for up to a year, depending on the circumstances. Table 14.1 outlines the recommendations for CNS and pulmonary infection in a case such as the one described here. Initial therapy includes amphotericin B (liposomal or lipid formulation) and usually flucytosine is included to treat CNS infection. It is important to monitor flucytosine levels. For consolidation and maintenance therapy, oral fluconazole, is usually recommended but the dose varies according to the disease.

Table 14.1 Outline of therapeutic approaches to treating cryptococcal infection in solid organ recipients

	Initial/Induction	Consolidation	Maintenance
Meningoencephalitis	Liposomal amphotericin B 3–4 m/kg/day + flucytosine 100 mg/kg/day × 2 weeks	Fluconazole 400–800/day x 8 weeks	Fluconazole 200–400 mg/day 6 months–1year
Pulmonary infection	Liposomal amphotericin B 3–4 mg/kg/day × 2 weeks	Fluconazole 400 mg/ day × 8 weeks	Fluconazole 200 mg/day for 6 months–1 year

Source: data from Skolnik K, Huston S, Mody CH, et al. (2017). Cryptococcal lung infections. *Clin Chest Med.* 38(3):451–464. Transmission of *Cryptococcus neoformans* by organ transplantation. *Clin Infect Dis.* 52(4):e94–e98.

14.8 Is it possible that this patient acquired the cryptococcal infection from the transplanted kidney?

No. The interval between transplantation and the presentation of cryptococcal infection—nine months—is too long. Cases of invasive cryptococcal infection have very occasionally been described in patients receiving organs from patients incubating the infection. However, infection in the transplanted patient usually presents within days or at most a few weeks after the transplant procedure. Organ donors with immunosuppressive disease or on immunosuppressive agents are at risk for onward transmission. However, currently, organ donors are not routinely screened for cryptococcal infection. Early cryptococcal infection after transplantation could also be due to the recipient incubating the undiagnosed infection at the time of transplantation, which then manifests with the use of immunosuppressive agents to prevent organ rejection.

Further reading

Skolnik K, Huston S, Mody CH. Cryptococcal lung infections. *Clin Chest Med* 2017; **38**: 451–464.

La Hoz RM, Pappas PG. Crytococcal Infections: Changing epidemiology and implications for therapy. *Drugs* 2013; **73**: 495–504.

Perfect JR, Bicanic T. Cryptococcosis diagnosis and treatment: what do we know now? *Fungal Gen Biol* 2015; **78**: 49–54.

Perfect JR, Dismukes WE, Dromer F, Goldman DL, Graybill JR, et al. Clinical Practice Guidelines for the Management of Cryptococcal disease: 2010 Update by the Infectious Diseases Society of America. *Clin Infect Dis* 2010; **50**: 291–332.

Baddley JW, Schain DC, Gupte A, Lodhi SA, Kayler LK, et al. Transmission of *Cryptococcus neoformans* by organ transplantation. *Clin Infect Dis* 2011; **52**: e94–e98.

Section 3

Gastrointestinal infections

Case 15

Hilary Humphreys

Case history

A 73-year-old man is admitted via the Emergency Department (ED) with an acute abdomen and sepsis. He had a myocardial infarction 5 years ago. He has otherwise been well and is only on a statin. On admission, he has a temperature of 39.5 °C, a blood pressure of 90/60 and a white cell count of 23×10^9L $(4-11 \times 10^9)$ with increased polymorph neutrophils. At laparotomy, a perforated colonic carcinoma is detected and there is generalized peritonitis. A colonic resection is undertaken and he returns to the intensive care unit for further management (Fig. 15.1).

Questions

15.1 How is this patient's peritonitis classified?

15.2 What empiric antibiotics might be used initially for this patient?

15.3 How important is empiric cover against enterococci?

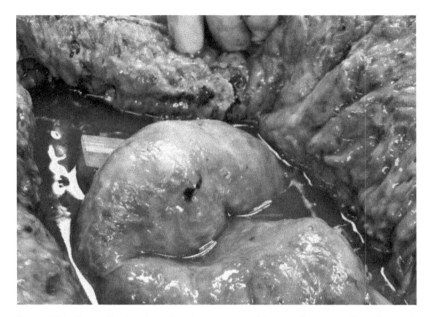

Figure 15.1 Generalized peritonitis at laparotomy with pus adherent to the colon and peritoneum (see colour plate).

Reproduced courtesy of Emma Tong, Royal College Surgeons in Ireland (RCSI), Ireland.

Answers

15.1 How is this patient's peritonitis classified?

Primary or spontaneous bacterial peritonitis is associated with ascites and significant liver disease and usually arises from translocation from the intestine. In adults, enteric bacteria are the most common cause but other causes such as *S. pneumoniae* may be responsible.

Secondary peritonitis arises from a perforated viscus as in the patient here and initial attempts at source control are important to control sepsis.

Peritonitis may also arise in the context of renal failure managed by continuous ambulatory peritoneal dialysis.

15.2 What empiric antibiotics might be used initially for this patient?

He needs broad-spectrum cover for aerobic Gram-negative bacilli and anaerobes. However, as he has been admitted from the community, has no immunosuppressive illness, and does not appear to have recently been admitted to hospital or received antibiotics, first-line agents may suffice. Therefore, co-amoxiclav or a second- or third-generation cephalosporin with metronidazole may be appropriate. The addition of metronidazole to co-amoxiclav is not usually necessary as the anaerobic cover with co-amoxiclav is usually adequate. However, increasing resistance to anti-anaerobic agents is being reported and susceptibility testing should be carried out on isolates if this is suspected on clinical grounds (e.g. the patient does not respond with apparent antibiotic cover) or if the patient has received prolonged courses of anti-anaerobic agents in the recent past. In the acutely septic patient, an aminoglycoside should be added initially to provide enhanced Gram-negative activity.

15.3 How important is empiric cover against enterococci?

The enterococci are considered less virulent than aerobic Gram-negative bacilli and for community-acquired intra-abdominal sepsis, enterococcal cover is not considered necessary. However, if operative or subsequent specimens are positive for enterococci or the patient remains septic, appropriate anti-enterococcal cover should be considered.

Case history continued

The patient is stabilized, started on intravenous co-amoxiclav and a dose of gentamicin, but remains ventilated and requires haemodynamic support. Blood cultures are negative but operative specimens grow *Escherichia coli* positive for extended-spectrum β-lactamases (ESBL). The intensivist requests advice on whether the antibiotic should be changed.

Questions

15.4 Should the patient remain on co-amoxiclav?

15.5 For how long does this patient need antibiotics?

Answers

15.4 Should the patient remain on co-amoxiclav?

In theory, the presence of a β-lactamase inhibitor in co-amoxiclav, that is, clavulanate, means that this antibiotic remains appropriate for infections caused by ESBL-positive bacteria. Recent changes in susceptibility testing in Europe and in the United States have suggested that the minimum inhibitory concentration is more important that the antibiotic resistance mechanism in guiding treatment choices. Nonetheless, conventional practice would not rely on a β-lactam/β-lactamase inhibitor combination in complex infections where isolates positive for β-lactamase are isolated. Small studies and reviews support the approach of changing from a β-lactam/β-lactamase combination. Therefore, alternatives in this patient would be

Table 15.1 Empiric antibiotic options to treat secondary peritonitis

Regimen	Spectrum	Comments
Amoxicillin + gentamicin + metronidazole	Enterococci, AGNB, anaerobes	Many AGNB are resistant to amoxicillin. Gentamicin is potentially toxic and does not penetrate into pus well but has good anti-AGNB activity.
Co-amoxiclav	Enterococci, AGNB, MSSA, anaerobes	Suitable in antibiotic naive patients from the community. Sometimes combined with an aminoglycoside. Metronidazole is sometimes recommended due to activity in acidic environments, e.g. pus.
Piperacillin-tazobactam	Enterococci, AGNB (including *Ps. aeruginosa*), MSSA, anaerobes	Greater coverage of AGNB, especially if infection is healthcare-associated.
Cephalosporin or ciprofloxacin + metronidazole	AGNB, anaerobes	Most cephalosporins (e.g. cefotaxime) lack activity against pseudomonas and all lack enterococcal activity. Risk for *C. difficile*.
Meropenem	Enterococci, AGNB, (including *Ps. aeruginosa* and ESBL producers), MSSA, anaerobes	Should be second-line unless ESBL+ve pathogens suspected.
Ceftolozane-tazobactam and ceftazidime-avibactam, both with metronidazole	Broad-spectrum but usually reserved for treating carbapenemase-producing Enterobacterales	Relatively new agents approved for complicated intra-abdominal infections, including for some ESBL infections and may have a role.

AGNB, aerobic Gram-negative bacilli, e.g. *E. coli*; MSSA, methicillin-susceptible *Staphylococcus aureus*; ESBL, extended-spectrum β-lactamase.

carbapenems such as meropenem, or a quinolone or an aminoglycoside with metronidazole. Options to cover peritonitis are outlined in Table 15.1.

15.5 For how long does this patient need antibiotics?

With adequate source control and an early resolution of clinical signs and symptoms, 5–7 days or fewer may be adequate, especially in patients not requiring organ support. However, critically ill patients who remain septic, especially if there are challenges in adequate source control, often remain on antibiotics for longer. The decision when to stop antibiotics is difficult in the acutely ill patient who remains pyrexial with elevated inflammatory markers. Consequently, the decision is often individualized according to the background and condition of the patient, and should be made by a multidisciplinary team (MDT) involving the surgeon, intensivist, and clinical microbiologist/infectious disease physician, amongst others. A balance has to be drawn between adequately treating the patient and minimizing antibiotic side effects and the emergence of resistance. If the patient fails to settle on appropriate antibiotics a persistent focus must be sought.

Case history continued

Over the course of the next 5 days, the patient remains pyrexial and continues to require haemodynamic support. Drains, inserted at laparotomy, are no longer draining pus or fluid. A computerized tomography (CT) scan of the abdomen and pelvis indicates a residual abscess.

Question

15.6 What are the options now for source control?

Answer

15.6 What are the options now for source control?

The decision as to whether to have an open procedure in the operating theatre or aspiration under radiological control is dependent upon the site of the abscess, its size, and the condition of the patient. Increasingly, drainage under radiological control is possible. However, this requires temporary transfer to the radiology department where this is normally undertaken under CT guidance. Therefore, the decision on what to do is usually made following discussions amongst the MDT. The procedure should result in adequate drainage, debridement, decompression, some restoration in anatomy and function, and specimens for culture to monitor if anti-infective cover is adequate, based on susceptibility testing.

Case history continued

Pus is aspirated at a repeat laparotomy, the patient settles, and he is eventually discharged to the ward for further management.

Question

15.7 How likely is surgical site infection after emergency bowel resection?

Answer

15.7 How likely is surgical site infection after emergency bowel resection?

Post-operative infection is very likely given an acute abdomen and an emergency laparotomy for a perforated viscus with generalized peritonitis. Up to a half of all patients in this setting develop post-operative infection, given the presence of peritonitis and significant contamination of the peritoneum, the skin, and associated structures. Microbial causes include aerobic Gram-negative bacilli, such as *E. coli* as well as *Pseudomonas aeruginosa* and *Candida* species.

Further reading

Ballus J, Lopez-Delgado JC, Sabater-Riera J, Perez-Fernandez XL, Betbese AJ, et al. Surgical site infection in critically ill patients with secondary and tertiary peritonitis: epidemiology, microbiology and influence in outcomes. *BMC Infect Dis* 2015; **15**: 304.

Harris PNA, Tambyah PA, Lye DC, Mo Y, Lee TH, et al. MERINO Trial Investigators and the Australasian Society for Infectious Disease Clinical Research Network (ASID-CRN). Effect of piperacillin-tazobactam vs meropenem on 30-day mortality for patients with *E coli* or *Klebsiella pneumoniae* bloodstream infection and ceftriaxone resistance: a randomized clinical trial. *JAMA* 2018; **320**: 984–94.

Lutz P, Nischalke HD, Strassburg CP, Spengler U. Spontaneous bacterial peritonitis: the clinical challenge of a leaky gut and cirrhotic liver. *World J Hepatol* 2015; **7**: 304–14.

Solomkin JS, Mazuski JE, Bradley JS, Rodvold KA, Goldstein EJ, et al. Diagnosis and management of complicated intra-abdominal infection in adults and children: Guidelines by the Surgical Infection Society and the Infectious Diseases Society of America. *Clin Infect Dis* 2010; **50**: 133–64.

Tamma PD, Rodriguez-Baño J. The use of noncarbapenem β-lactams for the treatment of extended-spectrum β-lactamase infections. *Clin Infect Dis* 2017; **64**: 972–80.

Case 16

Andrew Woodhouse

Case history

A 67-year-old man presents to hospital with a 5-day history of fever, chills, and vague right upper quadrant pain. He has type 2 diabetes mellitus, has recently been diagnosed with gallstones, and he has a 4-year history of diverticular disease. He was recently treated for an episode of abdominal pain and diarrhoea felt to be due to diverticulitis. He has a temperature of 38.5 °C, pulse of 120/minute, and is hypotensive (BP 95/60). His abdomen is soft but he has a palpable liver edge and is tender on deep palpation of his right upper quadrant. Blood tests show neutrophil leucocytosis, raised C-reactive protein (CRP) at 346 mg/L, and deranged liver enzyme tests in a cholestatic pattern with a normal bilirubin. His urine dip test is negative and a chest X-ray (CXR) is normal.

Questions

16.1 What immediate management is required?

16.2 What antibiotics should be started empirically?

Answers

16.1 What immediate management is required?

He has features of sepsis—a systemic inflammatory response due to an infection—in this case most likely bacterial. He needs evaluation for sepsis including lactate measurement, fluid resuscitation, oxygen, and antibiotics, initially started empirically based on the most likely source and administered promptly. He should have blood cultures taken, ideally two separate sets, and treatment started immediately. An intra-abdominal source seems highly probable and there is no evidence to support a urinary or respiratory tract origin.

16.2 What antibiotics should be started empirically?

The choice of empiric antibiotic will depend in part on local susceptibility patterns which should have informed the local guidelines. Prior to having initial imaging and microbiological results, a broad spectrum approach needs to be adopted with cover to include the Gram-negative enteric bacteria and intra-abdominal anaerobes. A broad-spectrum β-lactam/β-lactamase inhibitor combination is a reasonable choice (see Case 15). Although broad anaerobic coverage is a feature of these agents, some would advocate the addition of metronidazole to extend anaerobic activity further. A third-generation cephalosporin plus metronidazole is an option. In some environments the frequency of aerobic Gram-negative bacilli producing extended spectrum β-lactamases is such that initial treatment might be based on a carbapenem-containing regimen, again with or without metronidazole. All initial treatment needs to be reviewed in light of microbiological results as these become available.

Case history continued

He has an abdominal ultrasound which reports the presence of gallstones in a mildly oedematous gallbladder but no evidence of intra- or extra-hepatic duct dilatation. A hypoechoic lesion measuring 5 × 6 cm is seen in the right lobe of the liver and is felt to be consistent with a possible liver abscess. A computerized tomography (CT) scan is recommended to define the lesion further. The CT scan shows a single lesion in the right lobe and the radiologist feels the lesion is readily accessible for CT-guided drainage (Fig. 16.1).

Questions

16.3 What other information may be available from the CT scan relevant to the diagnosis?

16.4 When and how should liver abscesses be drained?

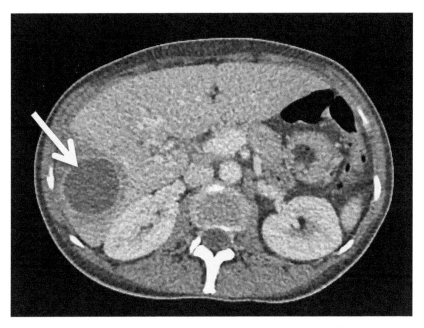

Figure 16.1 CT scan showing a liver abscess (arrow) in the right lobe of the liver.

Reproduced courtesy of University Hospitals Birmingham NHS Foundation Trust, UK.

Answers

16.3 What other information may be available from the CT scan relevant to the diagnosis?

The scan may show evidence of pathology which has predisposed to the development of the liver abscess. Diverticular disease is a risk factor for liver abscess and in the light of his history, a careful review to assess for evidence of ongoing diverticulitis or a cryptic diverticular abscess is important. Historically, appendicitis was a frequent association with liver abscess but it is unusual now. Previously undiagnosed inflammatory bowel disease is sometimes discovered in patients with liver abscess. Organisms gain access to the liver from distant abdominal foci via the portal vein as portal vein pyaemia and thrombosis of the portal vein may also be seen.

16.4 When and how should liver abscesses be drained?

In general, only very small liver abscesses are likely to respond to antimicrobial therapy alone without drainage. Radiology-guided aspiration and drainage has replaced surgical drainage in almost all situations. No absolute size cut-off for not draining has been defined but abscesses larger than 3 cm seem to do less well with antibiotics alone. Success with radiological drainage of large abscesses (> 10 cm diameter) is also increasingly reported. Surgery now tends to be reserved for non-responders or complex multiloculated collections. An indwelling drain should be used for larger abscesses but a small collection may be amenable to drainage via needle aspiration only. Obtaining pus for culture remains an important part of management even if blood cultures are positive as abscesses can be polymicrobial.

Case history continued

The CT scan also shows diverticular disease with appearances of the sigmoid colon consistent with diverticulitis. Admission blood cultures have grown *Klebsiella pneumoniae*. He has responded to fluids and antibiotics—amoxicillin/clavulanate and metronidazole—and he feels better but continues to have fevers. The organism is susceptible to the amoxicillin/clavulanate.

A drain is inserted into the abscess and material sent for culture grows *K. pneumoniae* and *E. faecalis*. Fluid continues to drain from the abscess for approximately 7 days but an ultrasound scan shows minimal residual fluid and the drain is removed at day 10.

Questions

16.5   What is the significance of the *Klebsiella pneumoniae* isolated in this context?

16.6   How long should antibiotics be continued?

Answers

16.5 What is the significance of the *Klebsiella pneumoniae* isolated in this context?

Klebsiella pneumoniae has been recognized as a cause of a primary invasive liver abscess syndrome in the absence of predisposing hepatobiliary or bowel disease. Most of the early reports of this condition were from Taiwan and other parts of South East Asia but other regions have subsequently observed a similar condition. Diabetes mellitus is the most commonly associated risk factor but the pathogenesis is not completely understood. Infection is almost always monomicrobial. In the case presented the presence of *K. pneumoniae* is unlikely to represent an example of this syndrome given the underlying bowel disease and polymicrobial culture.

16.6 How long should antibiotics be continued?

There is no evidence-based recommendation for duration of antibiotic treatment in liver abscess. Most suggestions and opinions are the result of experience and expert consensus. With adequate drainage most advice is to complete 4–6 weeks of antibiotic with parenteral therapy for perhaps the first half of treatment assuming a good clinical response. Follow-up imaging is recommended but imaging resolution is likely to lag behind clinical and microbiological cure.

Further reading

Heneghan HM, Healy NA, Martin ST, Ryan RS, Nolan N, et al. Modern management of pyogenic hepatic abscess: a case series and review of the literature. *BMC Research Notes* 2011; 4: 80.

Liao WI, Tsai S-H, Yu C-Y, Huang GS, Lin YY, et al. Pyogenic liver abscess treated by percutaneous catheter drainage: MDCT measurement for treatment outcome. *Eur J Radiol* 2012; 4: 609–15.

Mezhir JJ, Fong, Y, Jacks LM, Getrajdman GI, Brody LA, et al. Current management of pyogenic liver abscess: surgery is now second-line treatment. *J Am Coll Surg* 2010; 210: 975–83.

Mohsen AH, Green ST, Read RC, McKendrick MW. Liver abscess in adults: ten years experience in a UK centre. *QJM* 2002; 95: 797–802.

Siu LK, Yeh KM, Lin JC, Fung CP, Chang FY. *Klebsiella pneumoniae* liver abscess: a new invasive syndrome. *Lancet Infect Dis* 2012; 12: 881–7.

Case 17

Hilary Humphreys

Case history

A 57-year old female presents to her General Practitioner (GP) with a 3-day history of diarrhoea with 6 liquid stools a day. She had a recent urinary tract infection and completed a course of co-amoxiclav 7 days ago. She is not dehydrated, her abdomen is soft on examination, and her vital signs are normal. The GP considers *Clostridioides difficile* infection (CDI) in the differential diagnosis.

Questions

17.1 How do you classify diarrhoea arising in the community due to *C. difficile*?

17.2 Why is this patient not considered to have severe CDI?

17.3 What is the diagnostic test of choice for CDI?

Answers

17.1 How do you classify diarrhoea arising in the community due to *C. difficile?*

These are classified by the European Centre for Disease Control (ECDC) as follows:

◆ Healthcare-associated—symptoms on day 3 or later following admission to a healthcare facility on day 1, or onset of symptoms in the community but within 4 weeks of discharge from a healthcare facility.

◆ Community-associated—onset of symptoms outside healthcare facilities, without discharge from or being resident in a healthcare facility in the last 12 weeks.

◆ Unknown association—a case of CDI discharged from a healthcare facility 4–12 weeks before the onset of symptoms.[1]

17.2 Why is this patient not considered to have severe CDI?

Severe CDI is confirmed using clinical, laboratory, radiological, and endoscopic findings. There are a number of CDI severity scores which include leucocytosis ($> 15 \times 10^9$/L), elevated serum creatinine, ($> 50\%$ baseline), acute abdomen, ileus, fever > 38.5 °C high and megacolon, colonic wall thickening, or pericolonic fat stranding on computerized tomography (CT). Patients with severe ileus or colon wall oedema may not have diarrhoea.

17.3 What is the diagnostic test of choice for CDI?

Historically the diagnostic method was the detection of cytotoxin in cell lines from a diarrhoeal sample. Other methods now include detecting glutamate dehydrogenase (GDH) as a screening test followed by more specific immuno-assays (IA) for the detection of the toxins A and B in the stool, and/or toxin gene detection by PCR (Fig. 17.1). Whatever combination of tests are undertaken, they should include cytotoxin detection. Some molecular tests also detect the presence of binary toxin, a marker for virulence. The detection of *C. difficile* DNA by PCR does not confirm that toxin is being produced and a PCR-positive test may occur in patients without CDI. Therefore, the interpretation of positive PCR test results should be correlated with clinical features, and preferably with a second test (e.g. IA) to differentiate colonization from infection. The status of symptomatic patients who are PCR positive but IA negative is uncertain. These may subsequently become toxin positive and may transmit infection, if not isolated.

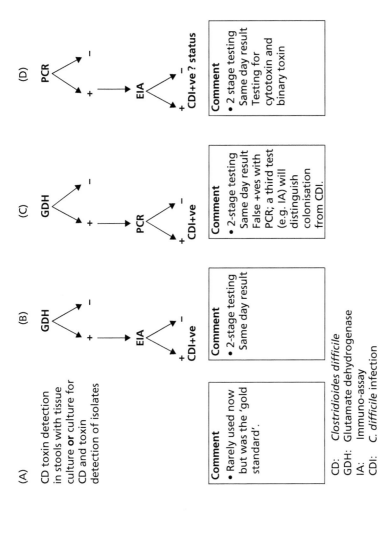

Figure 17.1 Diagnostic testing options.

Case history continued

The GP sends a stool sample to the local microbiology laboratory. Subsequently, CDI is confirmed by PCR and by IA. She prescribes an appropriate agent for 14 days and the symptoms resolve. However, 4 weeks after stopping CDI treatment, the patient develops another episode of diarrhoea and repeat testing confirms toxin-positive CDI.

Questions

17.4 What is the preferred management of this patient?

17.5 Is this second episode recurrent CDI or a new infection?

17.6 What are the options for the treatment of recurrent CDI?

17.7 What is the role of faecal microbiota transplantation (FMT)?

17.8 What is the treatment of severe complicated CDI?

Answers

17.4 What is the preferred management of this patient?

General measures include:

- Adequate nutrition, fluid, and electrolytes replacement
- Stop unnecessary antimicrobials
- Avoid anti-motility medications
- Patient isolation with contact precautions if in a healthcare facility

Mild disease may be treated by discontinuing any precipitating antimicrobials and rehydration. Specific treatment for ongoing symptomatic CDI is increasingly oral vancomycin for 10 days in preference to metronidazole, especially when there is an elevated white cell count or an elevated creatinine, or in older patients, or those with a more virulent strain. Vancomycin also has higher cure rates for severe disease.

17.5 Is this second episode recurrent CDI or a new infection?

This is recurrent CDI as the symptoms have recurred within 8 weeks after the onset of a previous episode. This occurs in 15–20% of patients.

17.6 What are the options for the treatment of recurrent CDI?

A first recurrence may be treated with oral vancomycin as a tapered and pulsed dose regimen, or with fidaxomicin (Table 17.1). Fidaxomicin is not effective for CDI due to ribotype 027. The indications for fidaxomicin in patients with recurrent CDI include adult patients with mild-to-moderate or severe CDI, and where concomitant antimicrobials need to be used. Fidaxomicin is a non-absorbable macrocyclic antibiotic and preserves the normal flora of the gastrointestinal tract better than many other antibiotics. Other options include rifaximin and nitazoxinide but these have not been extensively studied. The patient should also be observed closely for possible deterioration and their nutritional/hydration status reviewed.

17.7 What is the role of faecal microbiota transplantation (FMT)?

FMT may be administrated orally, via a naso-gastric tube, or rectally, and improves colonic microbial diversity with increases in *Bacteroides* spp. and *Firmicutes*, and decreased *Proteobacteria*. Randomized controlled trials show that symptoms resolve in ≥ 85% of cases but issues remain about screening donors of FMT and its optimal administration. This may become the therapeutic option of choice in the future for recurrent CDI.

Table 17.1 Therapeutic options for treating recurrent CDI

Therapy	Comment
Repeat initial therapy	Vancomycin preferred for subsequent recurrences
Tapered vancomycin over 2 weeks	Reduced dose interval from ×4/day to once every 72 hours over 2 weeks
Fidaxomicin	Lower recurrence rate if initial therapy (except ribotype 027) and preferred if other antibiotics can't be discontinued
Faecal microbiota transplantation	Effective in > 85% of patients
Monoclonal antibodies	Trials assessed efficacy as initial treatment in combination with antibiotics with reduced recurrence rate *vs.* antibiotics alone
Other Agents	Rifaximin, nitazoxinide, tigecycline, fuscidic acid, probiotics, toxin binders (e.g. colestipol), non-toxigenic *C.difficile*, intravenous immunoglobulin; anecdotal evidence, small studies or case reports only.

17.8 What is the treatment of severe complicated CDI?

Vancomycin administered orally or via a naso-gastric tube for up to 14 days is the treatment of choice and may also be administered rectally in the setting of ileus. Usually intravenous metronidazole is administered concomitantly to achieve detectable levels throughout the colon. However, early surgical evaluation and imaging are essential such as to diagnose megacolon, when subtotal colectomy with an end-ileostomy is required to reduce mortality.

Acknowledgements

Thanks to Fidelma Fitzpatrick.

Further reading

Bagdasarian N, Rao K, Malani PN. Diagnosis and treatment of *Clostridium difficile* in adults. a systematic review. *J Am Med Ass* 2015; **313**: 398–408.

Cammarota G, Ianiro G, Tilg H, Rajilić-Stojanović M, Kump P, et al. European consensus conference on faecal microbiota transplantation in clinical practice. *Gut* 2017; **66**: 569–80.

Chen S, Gu, H, Sun C, Wang H, Wang J. Rapid detection of *Clostridium difficile* toxins and laboratory diagnosis of *Clostridium difficile* infections. *Infection* 2017; **45**: 255–62.

European Centre for Disease Prevention and Control. European Surveillance of Clostridium difficile infections. Surveillance protocol version 2.3. Stockholm: ECDC; 2017. https://ecdc.europa.eu/sites/portal/files/documents/European-surveillance-clostridium-difficile-v2point3-FINAL_PDF3.pdf

McDonald LC, Gerding DN, Johnson S, Bakken JS, Carroll KC, et al. Clinical Practice guidelines for *Clostridium difficile* infection in adults and children: 2017 Update by the Infectious Diseases Society of America (IDSA) and Society for Healthcare Epidemiology of America (SHEA). *Clin Infect Dis* 2018; **66**: e1–e48.

Case 18

Andrew Woodhouse

Case history

A previously healthy 32-year-old man is referred because of diarrhoea which has persisted for 4 weeks after returning from a 4-week trip to Thailand where he travelled in rural areas in addition to a week at a beach resort. During the first week of his trip he experienced an acute illness with cramping abdominal pain and the passage of up to 6 watery motions per day with occasional sweats. A travelling companion gave him a 3-day course of ciprofloxacin together with loperamide and his diarrhoea settled over a 4-day period. He continued to take occasional loperamide until a week before he left Thailand but felt well. He noticed loose stools again during the last week of his trip but without abdominal pain. His symptoms have persisted and he continues to pass semi-liquid stools up to 3 times per day with occasional abdominal discomfort and belching, but there are no systemic symptoms. He is afebrile and clinical examination is normal apart from mild central abdominal tenderness.

Questions

18.1 What was his acute illness in Thailand?

18.2 Which microbes are most commonly associated with acute diarrhoea during travel?

18.3 What are the potential causes of his current symptoms and what investigations are indicated?

18.4 What treatment is indicated for this condition, and if so what agents would be appropriate?

18.5 What can be done to prevent this condition in travellers to resource-poor countries?

Answers

18.1 What was his acute illness in Thailand?

The acute onset of diarrhoea with abdominal pain in the context of travel to resource-poor countries suggests traveller's diarrhoea (TD). Diarrhoea is a common symptom among travellers with the risk varying depending on the region of the world visited. The highest risk destinations for TD include South and Central America, South and South East Asia, and Africa, other than South Africa. Most TD occurs early in the course of a trip, often within the first week of travel. The majority of episodes are short lived and last less than a week but depending on severity can impact adversely on holiday and business travel plans.

18.2 Which microbes are most commonly associated with acute diarrhoea during travel?

Studies of travel-related diarrhoea find no cause in up to 50% of cases but the commonest identified causes of TD are bacterial, with the diarrhoea-causing *E. coli* including enterotoxigenic *E. coli* (ETEC) and enteroaggregative *E. coli* (EAEC) responsible for the majority of episodes. *Campylobacter jejuni*, non-typhi *Salmonella* spp., and *Shigella* spp. are less frequent but important causes, particularly due to their potential to cause invasive disease. There is regional variation across the tropics with *C. jejuni*, for example, being the most common cause in South East Asia. Viral causes include norovirus, which is particularly notable for outbreaks on cruise ships. Parasites are relatively uncommon causes of TD but need to be considered in more chronic cases, especially giardia.

18.3 What are the potential causes of his current symptoms and what investigations are indicated?

Prolonged symptoms due to TD are rare. Persistence beyond 2 weeks occurs in only about 5% of patients. The history in this case suggests an initial acute improvement with subsequent ongoing less severe symptoms. A recurrence of the original illness is possible but an alternative pathogen should also be considered. A basic evaluation should include full blood count (FBC), inflammatory markers such as C-reactive protein (CRP), renal and liver function, and stool examination. The stool request should note the travel history and request culture and/or PCR for enteric pathogens and also evaluation for ova, cysts, and parasites. The use of PCR has superseded culture for common enteric pathogens in some centres with increased diagnostic sensitivity and shorter turnaround times. Giardia PCR is also more sensitive compared to stool microscopy in the diagnosis of giardiasis.

Giardiasis in particular should be considered given the chronicity of his current symptoms even though the original illness may have been bacterial. While unlikely,

Clostridiodies difficile infection should also be excluded given the recent empiric fluoroquinolone course.

A well-recognized entity to be aware of is a post-infectious irritable bowel syndrome following enteric infection. This is, however, a diagnosis of exclusion.

18.4 What treatment is indicated for this condition, and if so what agents would be appropriate?

Most cases of bacterial TD are relatively short lived, resolving over a matter of days, and don't require antibiotic treatment. Maintaining hydration is important and this should be emphasized to travellers. Clear fluids with sugar and ensuring dietary intake of salt (e.g. soups) is appropriate for healthy adults while oral rehydration solution may be needed for children or the elderly. Anti-motility agents such as loperamide have a role in controlling diarrhoea provided symptoms don't suggest invasive infection.

A number of studies and systematic reviews have shown a benefit from short courses of antibiotics compared to placebo with a reduction in the duration of illness from around 3 days to 1.5 days. This has led to standby courses of antibiotic being prescribed for travellers to self-administer, particularly those travelling to remote regions in high-risk countries or those likely to tolerate dehydration poorly. The choice of antibiotic is dependent on travel itinerary—for example, widespread fluoroquinolone resistance in South East Asia makes it less useful in that region than alternatives such as azithromycin. Rifamixin is a poorly absorbed rifamycin with efficacy in TD when compared to placebo but it is not recommended for invasive disease and has little activity against *Campylobacter* spp. Typical standby treatment courses are outlined in Table 18.1.

The use of antibiotics to treat TD is not without potential adverse consequences, including the acquisition of multi-resistant organisms, in particular extended spectrum β-lactamase-producing *Enterobacteriaciae* spp., and *C. difficile* infection.

Table 18.1 Standby treatment options for travellers' diarrhoea

Drug	Dose	Duration	Comment
Ciprofloxacin	750 mg	Single dose	Avoid in SE Asia where there are high rates of quinolone resistance.
	500 mg bd	3 days	
Azithromycin	1000 mg	Single dose	Most universally effective standby treatment.
	500 mg daily	3 days	
Rifaximin	200 mg 3× daily	3 days	Not recommended in invasive disease which limits its use as standby treatment.

If symptoms persist, such as in the case described, and other causes are excluded, a trial of nitroimadazole treatment such as metronidazole or tinidazole may be warranted for possible giardiasis, even if stool investigations are negative.

18.5 What can be done to prevent this condition in travellers to resource-poor countries?

Prevention of TD by hygiene measures and avoidance of high-risk foods and drinks is intuitive and should be discussed with travellers. However, the available evidence suggests a lack of effectiveness perhaps because it is not easy for travellers to judge risk accurately.

Prevention of TD by the use of daily antimicrobial agents (e.g. ciprofloxacin or rifaximin) as prophylaxis has been evaluated and been found to be effective compared to placebo but is not recommended for the majority of travellers. Prophylaxis may be appropriate in selected circumstances, such as immunocompromised or debilitated hosts where the consequences of severe illness may be significant. In addition short-term travellers with critical duties which preclude time off due to illness might also be considered for prophylaxis. As with all antibiotic treatment, the potential adverse effects of antibiotic exposure through prophylaxis including the acquisition of resistant organisms should be considered and discussed with the patient.

Further reading

Barett J, Rown M. Traveller's diarrhoea. *Br Med J* 2016; **353**: i1937. doi: 10.1136/bmj.i1937.

De Bruyn G, Hahn S, Borwick A. Antibiotic treatment for travellers' diarrhoea. *Cochrane Database Syst Rev* 2000; CD002242. Review.

Harvey K, Esposito DH, Han P, Kozarsky P, Freedman DO, et al. Centers for Disease Control and Prevention (CDC). Surveillance for travel-related disease—Geosentinel Surveillance System, United States, 1997–2011. *MMWR Surveill Summ* 2013; **62**: 1–23.

Kantele A, Lääveri T, Mero S, Vilkman K, Pakkanen SH, et al. Antimicrobials increase travelers' risk of colonization by extended-spectrum betalactamase-producing *Enterobacteriaceae*. *Clin Infect Dis* 2015; **60**: 837–46. doi:10.1093/cid/ciu957.

Steffen R, Hill DR, DuPont HL. Traveler's diarrhoea: a clinical review. *JAMA* 2015; **313**: 71–80. doi:10.1001/jama.2014.17006.

Case 19

T H Nicholas Wong

Case history

An 82-year-old man presents to the Emergency Department (ED) with a 24-hour history of nausea, vomiting, and diarrhoea. He has had 10 episodes of vomiting and approximately 20 episodes of watery diarrhoea since the illness began. This is associated with abdominal discomfort, generalized weakness, and headaches. Due to a lack of appetite and copious episodes of nausea, he is unable to eat and drink. He lives alone at home.

On examination, he is pyrexial (38.2 °C) and tachycardic (120 beats/min). Full blood count (FBC) as well as urea and electrolytes are within normal limits apart from hypokalaemia (2.8 mmol/L).

Questions

19.1 What organism is likely to have caused this?

19.2 Describe the epidemiology, impact, and transmission of this pathogen.

19.3 How can the causal agent be identified?

19.4 What is the treatment?

Answers

19.1 What organism is likely to have caused this?

The history suggests gastroenteritis. Given the headache and generalized malaise, this is most consistent with a viral gastroenteritis but other causes of infective gastro-enteritis must be considered (including *Clostridioides difficile*-associated diarrhoea if the patient has recently received antibiotics). The most common causes of viral gastroenteritis are caliciviruses (e.g. norovirus and sapovirus), rotavirus, astrovirus, and enteric adenoviruses (serotypes 40 and 41). Although this clinical presentation could be due to any of the viruses discussed previously, the most likely cause in adults will be norovirus.

Table 19.1 depicts the estimated number of cases of infectious intestinal disease (IID) in the community and presenting to general practice by organism in the United Kingdom, 2008–09. This was a UK longitudinal study involving symptomatic participants belonging to multiple general practices (GPs) that were followed up over a 1- year period. Stool specimens were tested from both symptomatic participants in the community (who did not present to their GP), as well as those who did present symptomatically to their GP.

19.2 Describe the epidemiology, impact, and transmission of this pathogen.

The family caliciviridae is divided into five genera: Lagovirus, Nobovirus, Norovirus, Sapovirus, and Vesirus. Noroviruses are single-stranded positive-sense RNA viruses. There are currently seven recognized genogroups based on sequence diversity in VP1, the major capsid protein. Within each genogroup there are multiple genotypes. GII.4 (genogroup 2, genotype 4) norovirus has been the predominant strain responsible for the majority of worldwide norovirus outbreaks in the last 15 years. Norovirus affects people of all ages and causes around 90% of non-bacterial acute gastroenteritis worldwide. It remains the primary cause of endemic diarrhoea in children.

Norovirus is estimated to cost the National Health Service over £100 million per annum in years of high incidence. Approximately 3,000 people each year are admitted to hospital with norovirus in England and the incidence in the community is thought to be about 17% of the 17 million cases of IID in England per year.

Transmission is faeco-oral, but contaminated surfaces and aerosolization during vomiting episodes have been reported. Norovirus can survive at a wide range of temperatures and is relatively resistant to simple detergents and common ethanol-based disinfectants. It is effectively killed by bleach. The infectious dose can be as low as 10–100 viral particles.

19.3 How can the causal agent be identified?

Individual cases do not normally require specific diagnostic testing as the diagnosis is based on clinical features and treatment is supportive. A number of commercial

Table 19.1 Estimated number of cases of infectious intestinal disease (IID) in the community and presenting to general practice by organism, Infectious Intestinal Disease 2 Study, UK 2008–9

Organism	Community cases (%)	GP presentation cases (%)
Bacteria		
C. perfringens	89,847 (0.53)	14,983 (1.37)
Campylobacter spp.	571,949 (3.38)	78,973 (7.2)
E. coli 0157 (VTEC)	18,916 (0.11)	824 (0.08)
Enteroaggressive *E coli*	365,297 (2.16)	12,893 (1.18)
Salmonella spp.	38,606 (0.23)	11,291 (1.03)
Protozoa		
Cryptosporidium	43,834 (0.26)	12,488 (1.14)
Giardia	52,434 (0.31)	5,617 (0.51)
Viruses		
Adenovirus	630,251 (3.72)	52,106 (4.75)
Astrovirus	325,642 (1.92)	24,982 (2.28)
Norovirus	2,905,278 (17.16)	128,022 (11.68)
Rotavirus	783,737 (4.63)	83,850 (7.65)
Sapovirus	1,610,041 (9.51)	97,024 (8.85)
All IID	16,935,420	1,096,190

Adapted with permission from Tam CC, et al. (2012). Longitudinal study of infectious intestinal disease in the UK (IID2 study): incidence in the community and presenting to general practice. *Gut.* 61(1):69–77. DOI: http://dx.doi.org/10.1136/gut.2011.238386

tests on stool samples have become available to detect both genogroup I and II disease. These incorporate an enzyme immuno-assay (EIA) but only have a sensitivity of around 58% with a specificity of 92%. RT-PCR remains the gold standard method for detection and has the greatest sensitivity. In addition, multiplex PCR faecal testing has also become available with the added benefits of detecting both bacterial and viral pathogens simultaneously.

19.4 What is the treatment?

Norovirus infection is usually self-limiting. Fluid and electrolyte correction remains the mainstay of treatment. Due to the difficulty of clearing the virus in the immuno-compromised, these patients may develop protracted diarrhoea, leading to dehydration and, in some cases, death. Diarrhoea is a common symptom in transplant recipients but testing for norovirus and other infectious agents should be considered in all cases when the cause is unclear.

Case history continued

Thirty-six hours after this patient was admitted, a patient within the bay develops symptoms of diarrhoea and vomiting. Twelve hours later a further 4 cases are reported within the ward, with 2 staff members absent due to similar symptoms.

Questions

19.5 What are the criteria for identifying an outbreak of viral gastroenteritis?

19.6 How should this scenario be managed?

Answers

19.5 What are the criteria for identifying an outbreak of viral gastroenteritis?

The Kaplan criteria can be applied during an outbreak to determine the probability of this being due to viral gastroenteritis. These criteria utilize four main predictors:

1. A mean (or median) illness duration of 12–60 hours;

2. A mean (or median) incubation period of 24–48 hours;

3. More than 50% of people with vomiting; and

4. No bacterial agent found.

These criteria have been associated with a sensitivity of around 70% and a specificity of up to 99%. The low sensitivity means norovirus cannot be excluded as the aetiological agent even if an outbreak fails to meet the criteria. Some norovirus outbreaks are predominantly diarrhoeal. Furthermore, additional cases may have resulted by the time both the incubation and illness duration have been met meaning that the Kaplan criteria can only be used retrospectively.

19.6 How should this scenario be managed?

Every hospital should have an infection prevention and control policy. Advice should be sought from the infection prevention and control team in all suspected outbreaks. Published guidelines from Public Health England (PHE) for ward management during a suspected outbreak are shown in Fig. 19.1. This includes closing affected bay(s) to admissions and transfers. Visitors who are symptomatic should not visit until 48 hours after the resolution of their symptoms. Non-essential visitors should be asked not to visit until the outbreak has ended. Essential visitors should be advised to take standard precautions on entering wards. Patients who need specialist treatment at other departments should be allowed to transfer but the receiving ward/departments must be informed and infection prevention and control preparations made. Staff need to be aware of affected patients and practise meticulous hand hygiene with soap and water before and after patient contact. Alcohol gels have been deemed not to be as effective as handwashing. Discharge of affected patients to nursing, residential homes, or other hospitals should be delayed until the patient has been asymptomatic for at least 48 hours. Affected ward staff should not return to work until they have been asymptomatic for 48 hours.

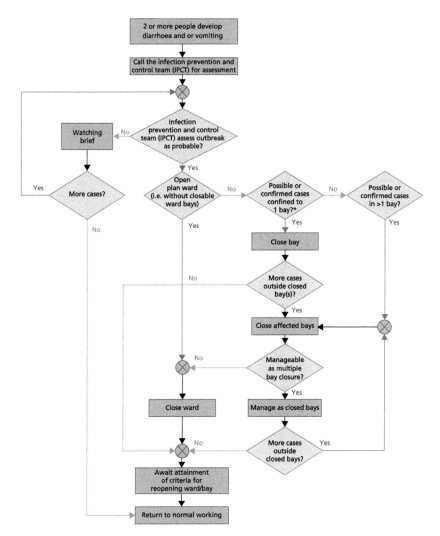

Figure 19.1 Algorithm for closure of bays or other clinical areas (see colour plate).

Reproduced with permission from Health Protection Scotland. (2013). *HPS Norovirus Outbreak Guidance: Preparedness, Control Measures, and Practical Considerations for Optimal Patient Safety and Service Continuation in Hospitals.* © Copyright Health Protection Scotland for the NHS National Services Scotland, the NHS Scotland and its agents.

Further reading

Guidelines for the management of norovirus outbreaks in acute and community health and social care settings. Produced by the Norovirus Working Party. Public Health England, 2012.

Kaplan JE, Feldman R, Campbell DS, Lookabaugh C, Gary GW. The frequency of a Norwalk-like pattern of illness in outbreaks of acute gastroenteritis. *Am J Public Health* 1982; **72**: 1329–32.

Lopman BA, Reacher MH, Vipond IB, Hill D, Perry C, et al. Epidemiology and cost of nosocomial gastroenteritis, Avon, England, 2002–2003. *Emerg Infect Dis* 2004; **10**: 1827–34.

Patel MM, Widdowson MA, Glass RI, Akazawa K, Vinje J, et al. Systematic literature review of role of noroviruses in sporadic gastroenteritis. *Emerg Infect Dis* 2008; **14**: 1224–31.

Tam CC, Rodrigues LC, Viviani L, Dodds JP, Evans MR, et al. Longitudinal study of infectious intestinal disease in the UK (IID2 study): incidence in the community and presenting to general practice. *Gut* 2012; **61**: 69–77.

Case 20

William L. Irving

Case history

A woman aged 41 received a third renal transplant, the first two having failed. She was well on follow-up but had a raised alanine aminotransferase (222 IU/ml, normal range 0–35) and aspartate aminotransferase (112 IU/ml, 0–30) on routine testing 4 years later. Liver function tests (LFTs) performed 3 months before this were normal. Repeat of her LFTs showed her alanine aminotransferase (ALT) and aspartate transaminase (AST) to be persistently raised over the next 12 months, although she remained well. She is referred to a hepatologist for assessment. Her immunosuppressive therapy comprises tacrolimus 4 mg od, mycophenolic acid 540 mg bd, and prednisolone 5 mg od. She is on a considerable number of other medications for co-morbidities, including cinacalcet, zopiclone, aspirin, lansoprazole, amlodipine, oxazepam, citalopram, ramipril, and simvastatin.

Questions

20.1 What causes of a raised ALT/AST should be considered and what investigations should be initiated?

20.2 The following results are reported. What is the diagnosis?

- Hepatitis B surface antigen: Negative
- Hepatitis B DNA: Negative
- Anti-HCV: Negative
- HCV RNA: Negative
- IgG anti-HEV: Negative
- IgM anti-HEV: Negative
- HEV RNA: Positive, viral load 2,200,000 IU/ml

20.3 What options are available to treat this infection?

20.4 How is HEV infection acquired, and how may it be prevented?

20.5 What complications are associated with HEV infection?

Answers

20.1 What causes of a raised ALT/AST should be considered and what investigations should be initiated?

The patient has presented with an apparently asymptomatic chronic transaminitis. The most likely cause is some form of chronic inflammatory hepatitis. Given the polypharmacy, drug-induced liver disease must be considered. Investigations should include an autoimmune screen, serum iron and ferritin, and a liver ultrasound. The important infections to consider are hepatitis B, C, and E viruses (HBV, HCV, HEV). Given that the patient is immunosuppressed, serological assays may not be informative, and therefore it is important to perform genome detection assays for HBV DNA, HCV RNA, and HEV RNA.

20.2 The following results are reported. What is the diagnosis?

- Hepatitis B surface antigen: Negative
- Hepatitis B DNA: Negative
- Anti-HCV: Negative
- HCV RNA: Negative
- IgG anti-HEV: Negative
- IgM anti-HEV: Negative
- HEV RNA: Positive, viral load 2,200,000 IU/ml

The presence of HEV RNA in a peripheral blood sample indicates current infection with HEV. The absence of detectable antibodies might indicate that this is a recent infection, but the immunosuppression may mean that the serology results are unreliable, and chronic HEV infection cannot be excluded at this stage. The laboratory retrieved several stored samples from this patient, confirming a diagnosis of chronic HEV infection in the absence of seroconversion (Table 20.1).

20.3 What options are available to treat this infection?

Chronic HEV infection is becoming an increasingly recognized condition in patients with significant immunosuppression such as a solid organ or bone marrow transplant recipient, HIV infection, and in some patients with underlying morbidities such as rheumatoid arthritis, inflammatory bowel disease, or sarcoidosis. Chronic infection is associated with a chronic inflammatory hepatitis which may progress rapidly to cirrhosis, hence the need for antiviral therapy.

The initial approach to management of chronic HEV infection in an immunocompromised patient is to try to reduce the level of immunosuppression. This results in viral clearance in around one-third of patients. If this fails or is not possible, then empirical therapy with a number of antiviral agents has been reported.

Table 20.1 Patient results

Sample number	Timing of sample in relation to presentation with abnormal LFTs	HEV IgM	HEV IgG	Plasma HEV viral load (IU/ml)	ALT (0–35 IU/ml)	AST (0–30 IU/ml)
1	3 months previously				25	30
2	At presentation	Neg	Neg	7.4×10^4	222	112
3	1 month later	Neg	Neg	2.2×10^6	167	96
4*	4 months later	Neg	Neg	Detected < 100	13	16
5*	6 months later	Neg	Neg	Detected < 100	14	18
6*	7 months later	Neg	Neg	Not detected	13	20
7*	8 months later	Pos	Neg	Detected <100	13	22
8*	9 months later	Pos	Neg	Not detected	15	21
9	11 months later			4.4×10^4	12	24
10	12 months later			3.2×10^4	22	22
11	21 months later				159	85

* The patient received ribavirin therapy.

The most successful is undoubtedly ribavirin, although the precise mechanism of action is unknown. In a large, retrospective study of nearly 60 patients treated with oral ribavirin for 3 months (median dose 600 mg/day), sustained viral clearance was achieved in 80% of patients. Treatment failure was associated with a low lymphocyte count at the start of therapy and, most importantly, the persistence of viral excretion in stool at the end of therapy, even if plasma viraemia was undetectable. Thus, management should include HEV RNA testing in plasma and stool at the end of 3 months therapy, and if either is positive, therapy should be extended to 6 months. There is anecdotal evidence that 6 months retreatment with ribavirin may succeed in patients who fail an initial 3-month course. Options for patients who remain viraemic despite this are difficult. Some success has been reported with the use of interferon alpha in liver transplant recipients with chronic HEV infection, but this increases the risk of rejection in all organ-transplant settings. There are *in vitro* data suggesting that sofosbuvir, a drug developed as an inhibitor of HCV RNA polymerase, may inhibit HEV replication, but the very few case reports of clinical use of this agent, even combined with ribavirin, are not encouraging.

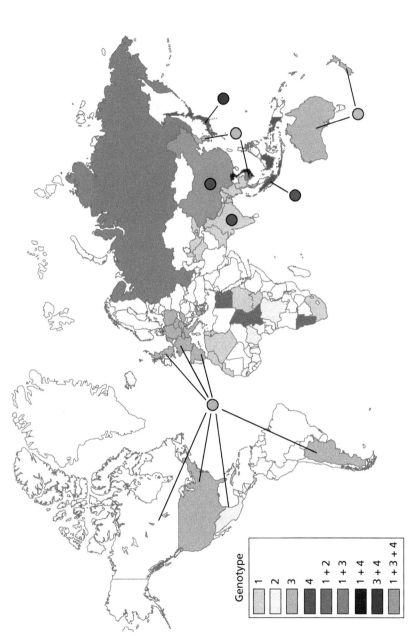

Figure 20.1 Distribution of HEV genotypes in viral isolates obtained from humans and animals (predominantly pigs). The colours used for a country and the circle associated with it represent the predominant HEV genotypes of human and animal isolates, respectively, from that country (see colour plate).

Reproduced with permission from Aggarwal. R. and Jameel, S. (2011). Hepatitis E. *Hepatology.* 54(6):2218–2226. DOI: 10.1002/hep.24674. *Source:* data from Okamoto, H. Genetic variability and evolution of hepatitis E virus. *Virus Res.* 127(2):216–228.

20.4 How is HEV infection acquired, and how may it be prevented?

Hepatitis E infection occurs globally, but there are virological and clinical differences depending on geography (see Fig. 20.1). In resource-poor countries, infection is with genotypes 1 and 2, which are spread faecal-orally, resulting in very high acute infection rates especially from faecal contamination of water supplies. In resource-rich countries, infection is usually with genotypes 3 and 4, and evidence is accumulating that these are zoonotic infections.

In the United Kingdom, infection in pigs is very widespread, with the swine virus being almost identical to human genotype 3 viruses. Thus, infection arises from consuming insufficiently cooked meat, predominantly processed pork meat.

Given that HEV must reach the liver via bloodstream spread, transmission via receipt of blood/blood products from viraemic donors is possible. Studies in a number of countries, including the United Kingdom, have revealed surprisingly high rates of HEV viraemia in blood donors—between 1 in 1,000 and 1 in 10,000 donors. Extrapolation of these data suggest that there must be up to 100,000 cases of acute HEV infection per year in the United Kingdom, almost all asymptomatic, and a small minority presenting with acute hepatitis.

There are a number of preventative strategies.

1. Travellers should be aware of possible contamination of water, and take appropriate precautions when abroad.

2. Within the United Kingdom, dietary risk is paramount, and therefore consumers of pork products should be educated to ensure adequate cooking—HEV has a high thermal stability, requiring temperatures of over 70 °C for inactivation. This advice is especially relevant to immunosuppressed transplant recipients (although abstinence would be even safer).

3. In view of the transfusion risks, many countries, including the United Kingdom, now screen all blood and organ donors for evidence of viraemia.

4. A number of vaccines have been trialled, the most promising being a recombinant peptide vaccine, shown to be effective in healthy Chinese adults, with a 3-dose regimen generating a durable antibody response in around 90% of those vaccinated. This vaccine is currently licensed for use and is available in China, but not elsewhere.

20.5 What complications are associated with HEV infection?

Acute infection may result in fulminant hepatitis, particularly in pregnant women in the third trimester who are infected with genotype 1 or 2 HEV. The mortality may be as high as 25%, although the pathophysiological reasons underlying this are not understood. Chronic infection in the immunocompromised is associated with progressive hepatitis and the development of cirrhosis.

A number of extrahepatic complications of HEV infection have been described, although a causal link has not always been established. These include neurological and renal complications, and acute pancreatitis occurring within 3 weeks of hepatitis onset. Neurological manifestations include Guillain–Barre syndrome (up to 5% of cases), neuralgic amyotrophy (also known as Parsonage–Turner syndrome or acute brachial neuropathy; HEV is associated with over 10% of such cases), meningoencephalitis, mononeuritis multiplex, and Bell's palsy. In support of these associations, HEV replicates *in vitro* in neuronal cells, and HEV RNA has been detected in the cerebrospinal fluid (CSF) of patients with these conditions. Renal manifestations include membranoproliferative glomerulonephritis, membranous nephropathy, and IgA (immunoglobulin A) nephropathy. Supportive evidence includes the identification of HEV RNA and HEV antigens in the urine of patients, and an increased HEV seroprevalence in haemodialysis patients, suggesting the possibility of HEV-induced glomerulonephritis leading to end-stage kidney disease. In addition, there are suggestions that HEV might also be associated with a range of other syndromes, including cryoglobulinaemia, thrombocytopaenia, monoclonal gammopathy of uncertain significance, arthritis, autoimmune thyroiditis, and myocarditis.

Further reading

Ankcorn MJ, Tedder RS. Hepatitis E: the current state of play. *Transfus Med* 2017; **27**: 84–95.

Arends JE, Ghisetti V, Irving W, Dalton HR, Izopet J, et al. Hepatitis E: an emerging infection in high income countries. *J Clin Virol* 2014; **59**: 81–8.

Dalton HR, Kamar N. Treatment of hepatitis E virus. *Curr Op Infect Dis* 2016; **29**: 639–44.

Pischke S, Hartl J, Pas SD, Lohse AW, Jacobs BC, et al. Hepatitis E virus: infection beyond the liver? *J Hepatol* 2017; **66**: 1082–95.

Case 21

William L. Irving

Case history

A 45-year-old man attends his General Practitioner (GP) for a health insurance check-up. He is well, with no significant past medical history. Clinical examination is unremarkable. Routine blood tests as required by the insurance company are sent to the laboratory. A week later, the patient is asked to revisit his GP as his blood tests have shown an elevated alanine aminotransferase (ALT) of 73 U/L (normal range 0–45) and an aspartate aminotransferase (AST) of 54 U/L (normal range 0–35). Other liver function tests are normal.

Questions

21.1 What further medical history should now be sought, and what further investigations conducted?

21.2 The GP receives the following results. What further actions should now be taken?

  - Hepatitis B surface antigen: Negative
  - Anti-HCV: Positive
  - HCV RNA: Positive, viral load 3.1×10^4 IU/ml

21.3 What drugs are available for treatment of this infection?

21.4 How is the success or otherwise of therapy measured?

21.5 What factors influence the response to therapy?

21.6 How should the patient be treated?

Answers

21.1 What further medical history should now be sought, and what further investigations conducted?

There are many causes of isolated raised transaminases, the most common being alcoholic liver disease, non-alcoholic fatty liver disease (NAFLD), and chronic viral hepatitis. The patient should be asked specific questions in his medical history including alcohol intake, recreational and medically prescribed drug use, sexual history, and family history of chronic hepatitis. Raised body mass index, and any other components of the metabolic syndrome (hypertension, glucose intolerance) would suggest NAFLD as a likely cause. Blood should be sent for hepatitis B and C (HBV, HCV) diagnostic testing.

21.2 The GP receives the following results. What further actions should now be taken?

- Hepatitis B surface antigen: Negative
- Anti-HCV: Positive
- HCV RNA: Positive, viral load 3.1×10^4 IU/ml

These results indicate current infection with HCV. The patient should be referred for specialist assessment, which will include viral genotyping and assessment of underlying liver damage. The latter is most commonly done using non-invasive tests such as transient elastography (also known as Fibroscan) or serum markers of fibrosis such as Fib4, APRI (aspartate aminotransferase to platelet ratio index) or ELF (enhanced liver fibrosis) tests. This is to determine whether or not the patient has cirrhosis.

21.3 What drugs are available for treatment of this infection?

In 1989, when the virus was first identified, the only option for therapy was standard interferon (IFN) given by subcutaneous injection thrice weekly. Improved response rates were seen with the introduction of pegylated IFN (PEG-IFN, given once weekly) in 1999, and then again with combination therapy of PEG-IFN plus ribavirin (RBV), which became the standard of care from 2001. The precise modes of action of either of these drugs are not known, but most likely they involve both antiviral effects and modulation of the host immune response to infection. A greater understanding of the molecular biology of the virus led to the identification of potential drug targets within the viral replication cycle, which in turn generated an avalanche of direct-acting antiviral agents (DAAs) entering clinical trials, initially in combination with PEG-IFN and RBV, but more recently, in interferon-free all-oral regimens. Whilst some of these DAAs fell by the wayside (mostly due to toxicity), some have demonstrated astounding success in eliminating HCV infection.

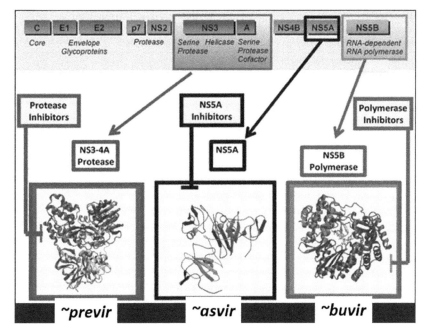

Figure 21.1 Hepatitis C virus (HCV) genome and potential drug discovery targets. The HCV RNA genome serves as a template for viral replication and as a viral messenger RNA for viral production. It is translated into a polyprotein that is cleaved by proteases. All the HCV enzymes—NS2- 3 and NS3-4A proteases, NS3 helicase, and NS5B RdRp— are essential for HCV replication, and are therefore potential drug discovery targets (see colour plate).

Adapted with permission from Asselah T and Marcellin P (2012). Direct acting antivirals for the treatment of chronic hepatitis C: one pill a day for tomorrow. *Liver Int.* 32 (Suppl 1):88–102. DOI: https://doi.org/10.1111/j.1478-3231.2011.02699.x.

Currently used DAAs fall into 3 categories, according to the viral target which they inhibit (see Fig. 21.1 and Table 21.1).

1. The NS3 protein (NS = non-structural). This molecule (with NS4A as a co-factor) has both protease and helicase activity. Drugs which inhibit this activity, known as protease inhibitors (PIs), carry the suffix –previr.

2. The NS5A protein. This multifunctional protein plays a number of key roles in the viral replication cycle, and in assembly and release of new viral particles. Drugs which inhibit this protein carry the suffix—asvir.

3. The NS5B protein. This is the RNA-dependent RNA polymerase (RdRp) enzyme. As is the case with anti-retroviral drugs, drugs which inhibit this viral polymerase may be nucleos(t)ide or non-nucleoside analogues. These drugs all carry the suffix—buvir.

Table 21.1 Direct-acting antiviral agents for the treatment of HCV infection

Viral target	Drugs	Comments
NS3/4A	Telaprevir, Boceprevir	First-wave first-generation drugs, now no longer used
	Simeprevir, Faldaprevir, Paritaprevir, Asunaprevir	Second-wave first-generation drugs, more potent, less toxic than first-wave drugs
	Grazoprevir, Voxelaprevir, Glecaprevir	Second-generation drugs, more pan-genotypic
NS5A	Daclatasvir, Ledipasvir, Ombitasvir, Velpatasvir, Pibrentasvir, Elbasvir, Ruzasvir*	
NS5B	Sofosbuvir, Uprifosbuvir*	Nucleos(t)ide analogues
	Dasabuvir	Non-nucleoside analogue

* Not currently licensed for use in the United Kingdom.

21.4 How is the success or otherwise of therapy measured?

The aim of therapy is to clear virus from the patient's peripheral blood (and by implication, liver). This is monitored by serial HCV RNA tests. The majority of patients achieve HCV RNA negativity by 4 weeks on therapy. Cessation of therapy may be accompanied by recrudescence of viraemia (responder–relapser), hence there is a need to continue monitoring after the end of treatment (EOT). Virological cure is now defined as being HCV RNA negative 12 weeks after EOT—this is termed a sustained virological response, or SVR12.

21.5 What factors influence the response to therapy?

There are several host and viral factors which impact on the rates of SVR12 associated with different therapeutic regimens.

Underlying liver damage

This is a key factor. Many trials show lower SVR12 rates in cirrhotic, as opposed to non-cirrhotic patients, and in decompensated versus compensated cirrhosis. Whilst the underlying reason for this is not clear (but may be due to inability of drugs to reach all infected hepatocytes in adequate concentration in a cirrhotic liver), the consequence of this observation is straightforward—regimens for treating cirrhotic patients are usually longer than for non-cirrhotics (e.g. for DAAs, 12 weeks as opposed to 8 weeks), and for some of the DAA regimens, it is recommended to add RBV for cirrhotic patients, especially if decompensated.

HIV co-infection

There is less chance of achieving SVR using IFN-based regimens, but in the DAA era, this is no longer the case. There is no need to institute different therapeutic regimens in HCV mono- and co-infected patients.

Compliance

This is a further and perhaps obvious host factor, but was of critical importance in the days of PEG-IFN/RBV therapy, as that combination was required for at least 6 months, and was associated with considerable morbidity, meaning that many patients were unable to tolerate taking a complete course of therapy.

Genotype

This is a reflection of the genetic variability of the virus (HCV genotypes are defined as having > 30% difference in nucleotide sequence across the whole genome). Genotypes 2 and 3 viruses are much more sensitive to the effects of IFN (SVR rates to PEG-IFN/RBV of the order of 75%), compared to genotype 1 (50%). Intergenotypic differences in the structure of the NS3 and NS5A proteins in particular mean that some of the DAA drugs are genotype (or even subtype) specific; for example, all the first-generation PIs had useful clinical activity only against genotype 1 viruses. Genotyping of an individual patient is an essential prerequisite to enable choice of the optimal treatment regimen. This problem is being overcome with the emergence of later generation DAAs which are more pan-genotypic in their activity.

Viral load

This was a useful predictor of response in the IFN era, but less so with the DAAs, although there is some evidence that patients with extremely high viral loads (i.e. in excess of 6×10^6 IU/ml) are less likely to achieve SVR.

Antiviral resistance

There is increasing recognition of the importance of resistance-associated substitutions (RAS) within the viral genome. Some of these are natural polymorphisms in circulating wild-type viruses—hence the term 'substitution' rather than 'mutation'. The barrier to development of resistance, and the degree of resistance conferred by each RAS varies, with the NS3/4A protease inhibitors (PIs) having the lowest barrier, and the nucleos(t)ide analogue NS5B inhibitors the highest.

21.5 How should the patient be treated?

The principles of treatment of chronic HCV infection are the same as for HIV, use of combinations of drugs acting on different viral targets (so as to minimize the possibility of emergence of fully resistant virus). Ideally, they should be given as simply as possible (i.e. 1 tablet a day) for as short a period of time as is compatible with cure.

Each pharmaceutical company manufacturing DAAs owns a number of different agents, and many of these are co-formulated into single tablets such as:

- Sofosbuvir + ledipasvir (Harvoni)
- Grazoprevir + elbasvir (Zepatier)
- Sofosbuvir + velpatasvir (Epclusa)
- Paritaprevir + ombitasvir + low-dose ritonavir (Viekirax)
- Glecaprevir + pibrentasvir (Maviret)
- Sofosbuvir + velpatasvir + voxelaprevir (Vosevi)

Treatment with any of these DAA regimens results in SVR12 rates in excess of 95% in almost all patient groups, the only exception being cirrhotic patients with genotype 3 infection who have failed previous therapy, where the rate is closer to 90%. Most regimens are for 12 weeks, but in some patient groups—for example, treatment-naïve non-cirrhotic genotype 1 infection—then 8 weeks may be sufficient. The extremely high cure rates associated with DAA therapy mean that resistance testing is not currently recommended for patients undergoing their first DAA regimen. The place of resistance testing in delineating optimal retreatment strategies for patients who fail DAA therapy has yet to be determined.

Further reading

AASLD-IDSA HCV Guidance Panel. Hepatitis C Guidance 2018 Update: AASLD-IDSA recommendations for testing, managing, and treating hepatitis C virus infection. *Clin Infect Dis* 2018; **67**: 1477–92.
EASL recommendations on treatment of hepatitis C. *J Hepatol* 2017; **66**: 153–94.

Section 4

Genitourinary infections

Case 22

Maheshi Ramasamy

Case history

A 33-year-old lady presents to the Emergency Department (ED) with a 3-day history of fever and back pain. She denies dysuria or frequency. She has type 1 diabetes mellitus and is on a continuous subcutaneous insulin pump. Her blood sugars have been increasingly erratic over the past 24 hours. On examination, she is alert and clinically dehydrated. She has a fever of 39.2 °C, a pulse rate of 110 beats per minute, and a blood pressure of 90/55. She has right flank tenderness to palpation. A clinical diagnosis of presumptive pyelonephritis is made.

Questions

22.1 What initial investigations should be performed?

22.2 What initial antibiotic therapy should be given and for how long?

22.3 Which patients require imaging and what is the ideal mode?

Answers

22.1 What initial investigations should be performed?

Significant pyuria is present in almost all patients with pyelonephritis and can be detected rapidly with bedside leukocyte esterase (sensitivity: 74–96% and specificity: 94–98%) and nitrite test (sensitivity: 35–85% and specificity: 92–100%). Microscopy is an alternative. A midstream urine should be sent for culture and susceptibility testing. Bacterial growth of > 10^5/ml colony-forming units on urine culture of a mid-stream specimen confirms the diagnosis. However, both pyuria and bacteriuria may be absent if the renal collecting system is obstructed and the infected focus does not communicate with the collecting system. Blood cultures should be done. A pregnancy test should be offered.

22.2 What initial antibiotic therapy should be given and for how long?

The most frequently isolated organism in pyelonephritis is *Escherichia coli* (Table 22.1). Patients with diabetes mellitus in particular are at risk of less common organisms such as *Klebsiella* spp., *Enterobacter* spp., or *Candida* spp. *Proteus* spp. are commonly associated with nephrolithiasis and identification of this organism in cultures should prompt investigation for renal calculi (see Question 22.3). The incidence of drug-resistant organisms varies between geographical location and empiric regimens should take local resistance patterns into consideration. Recent hospitalization, previous use of antibiotics, and immunosuppression are independent predictors of the prevalence of drug-resistant pathogens, in particular extended spectrum β-lactamase- (ESBL) producing organisms.

Table 22.1 Relative frequency (% of total) of bacterial species causing pyelonephritis

Organism	Frequency (%)
Escherichia coli	67
Klebsiella spp.	7.9
Proteus spp.	6.1
Enterobacter spp.	3.6
Enterococcus faecalis	3.4

Adapted from Buonaiuto VA, et al. (2014). Clinical and epidemiological features and prognosis of complicated pyelonephritis: a prospective observational single hospital-based study. *BMC Infect Dis*. 14: 639. Distributed under Creative Commons Attribution 4.0 International (CC BY 4.0).

Table 22.2 Risk factors associated with serious complications of pyelonephritis

Complication	Risk factors
Increased risk of death from pyelonephritis	◆ Age > 65 years ◆ Bedridden status ◆ Septic shock ◆ Recurrent acute pyelonephritis ◆ Diabetes mellitus ◆ Nephrolithiasis ◆ Immunosuppression
Prolonged hospitalization	◆ Diabetes mellitus ◆ Long-term urinary catheter ◆ Age > 65 years
Treatment failure	◆ Recent hospitalization ◆ Recent use of antibiotics

Source: data from Efstathiou, SP, et al. (2003). Acute pyelonephritis in adults: prediction of mortality and failure of treatment. *Arch In Med.* 163(10): 1206–1212. DOI:10.1001/archinte.163.10.1206.

Patients without sepsis or without risk factors for developing complications (Table 22.2) may be managed in the community with oral antibiotics. Possible regimens include an oral β-lactam/β-lactamase combination (co-amoxiclav), an oral cephalosporin, co-trimoxazole or a quinolone. If intravenous antibiotics are available in the community such as via an out-patient parenteral antibiotic therapy (OPAT) programme, then an intravenous cephalosporin (e.g. once daily ceftriaxone) or an aminoglycoside (gentamicin) can be considered for initial therapy in patients who are more unwell or have risk factors for more severe infections. In view of the risk of nephro- and oto- toxicity, aminoglycosides should be used with caution especially in those with renal impairment. The duration of aminoglycoside therapy should be limited where possible to 24–48 hours. For patients with known colonization with, or infection due to, ESBL-producing organisms, treatment should be based on known susceptibilities. Agents such as an intravenous carbapenem (ertapenem) may be required in some cases. Guidelines generally suggest treatment should be continued for 7 days, or 14 days if a β-lactam is used.

If the patient is hospitalized, the initial intravenous treatment should include a β- lactam/β-lactamase combination or a cephalosporin or a fluoroquinolone and/ or an aminoglycoside.

All antimicrobials should be used on the basis of local and national antibiotic guidelines and subsequent antibiotic susceptibility results.

22.3 Which patients require imaging and what is the ideal mode?

Imaging should be considered if the diagnosis is in doubt. The National Institute for Health and Care Excellence (NICE) guidance in the United Kingdom also recommends renal tract imaging to look for anatomical abnormalities of the renal tract in all male patients with pyelonephritis, all female patients following two or more episodes of pyelonephritis, and in all patients with *Proteus* spp. isolated in urine. A renal ultrasonography scan (USS) may be performed in the first instance to look for hydronephrosis or renal fat stranding. However, the sensitivity of computerized tomography (CT) or magnetic resonance imaging (MRI) is greater for detecting calculi, minor structural abnormalities, and renal abscesses (Fig. 22.1). CT is also superior to both intravenous urograms and USS in detecting renal parenchymal abnormalities such as perinephric stranding, decreased or delayed cortical enhancement, kidney enlargement, or gas formation, all of which may indicate more severe pyelonephritis. However, the contrast medium for CT imaging may cause an increase in serum creatinine in patients with renal failure. Pre-hydration of patients with intravenous fluids prior to administration of contrast can reduce the risk of contrast-induced nephropathy

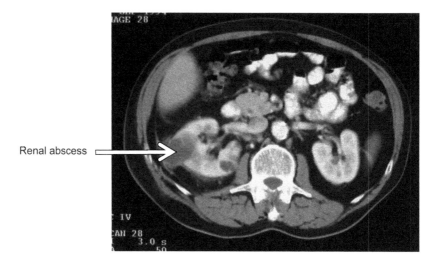

Renal abscess

Figure 22.1 CT image showing right perinephric abscess (arrow).

Reproduced courtesy of Philip J. Haslam, Newcastle upon Tyne Hospitals NHS Foundation Trust, UK.

Case history continued

The patient has a creatinine of 132 µmol/L on initial bloods and an estimated glomerular filtration rate of 45 ml/min. A pregnancy test is negative. She is treated with intravenous (IV) co-amoxiclav and has an ultrasound of her abdomen. This shows no obstruction and some inflammatory changes around her right kidney consistent with pyelonephritis. Blood cultures flag with a Gram-negative rod. The urine sample is also positive on culture. Preliminary identification and susceptibilities on each sample show an *Escherichia coli* susceptible to co-amoxiclav and gentamicin. The patient's pulse and blood pressure initially respond to intravenous fluids, but she continues to spike further temperatures. Thirty-six hours after admission, she becomes confused, profoundly hypotensive, and shocked.

Question

22.4   What would you do if the patient fails to respond despite appropriate anti-microbial therapy?

Answer

22.4 What would you do if the patient fails to respond despite appropriate antimicrobial therapy?

Patients with pre-existing structural or functional urinary tract abnormalities are more prone to pyelonephritis that is refractory to empirical treatment. Progressive symptoms in the context of a susceptible organism, as with this patient, should prompt further imaging to look for urinary tract abnormalities, an obstructed tract, a perinephric abscess that requires drainage, or nephrolithiasis. A specific consideration is emphysematous pyelonephritis, a rare but severe necrotizing multifocal pyelonephritis with gas formation visible on CT scanning. Treatment involves percutaneous drainage or nephrectomy.

Further reading

Buonaiuto VA, Marquez I, De Toro I, Joya C, Ruiz-Mesa JD, et al. Clinical and epidemiological features and prognosis of complicated pyelonephritis: a prospective observational single hospital-based study. *BMC Infect Dis.* 2014; **14**: 639. doi: 10.1186/s12879-014-0639-4.

Efstathiou SP, Pefanis AV, Tsioulos DI, Zacharos ID, Tsiakou AG, et al. Acute pyelonephritis in adults: prediction of mortality and failure of treatment. *Arch In Med* 2003; **163**: 1206–12.

Gupta K, Hooton TM, Naber KG, Wullt B, Colgan R, et al. Infectious Diseases Society of America; European Society for Microbiology and Infectious Diseases. International clinical practice guidelines for the treatment of acute uncomplicated cystitis and pyelonephritis in women: A 2010 update by the Infectious Diseases Society of America and the European Society for Microbiology and Infectious Diseases. *Clin Infect Dis* 2011; **52**: e103–20. doi: 10.1093/cid/ciq257.

National Institute for Health and Care Excellence. Knowledge Summary: Pyelonephritis [Internet] London UK: NICE; 2013 [updated June 2013; cited August 2017]. Available at: https://cks.nice.org.uk/pyelonephritis-acute#!topicsummary.

Neumann I and Moore P. Pyelonephritis (acute) in non-pregnant women *Br Med J Clin Evid* [Internet] 2014 Nov [cited 2017 Aug 05]; 2014: 0807. Available from: https://www.ncbi.nlm.nih.gov/pmc/articles/PMC4220693/.

Case 23

Hilary Humphreys

Case history

A 45-year-old male is on continuous ambulatory peritoneal dialysis (CAPD) for chronic renal failure. During the last 24 hours, he has noted that the dialysis fluid is cloudy and he has had some abdominal pain. A sample of CAPD fluid is sent to the microbiology laboratory and empirical antibiotics are commenced.

Questions

23.1 What is the most likely cause of this infection?

23.2 What criteria are used to confirm a microbiological diagnosis of infection?

23.3 What empirical antibiotics might this patient receive?

23.4 Why is intraperitoneal dosing usually preferred to intravenous dosing?

Answers

23.1 What is the most likely cause of this infection?

More than half of CAPD infections are due to Gram-positive organisms, specifically staphylococci, with coagulase negative staphylococci being more common than *Staphylococcus aureus*. Other causes include Gram-negative organisms, and occasionally fungi and mycobacteria. About one in five cases is culture negative.

23.2 What criteria are used to confirm a microbiological diagnosis of infection?

Usually there is a cell count of at least $100/mm^3$ or more in the CAPD fluid and at least 50% of these are polymorphs, assuming the fluid has been in the abdomen for more than 2 hours. In addition to direct culture, many CAPD samples are injected into blood culture bottles, which are then incubated as a blood culture, and then processed as such. This facilitates earlier culture positive results. Recent microbiology developments include improvements in organism identification and the use of molecular techniques to reduce the time to confirmation of infection.

23.3 What empirical antibiotics might this patient receive?

Antibiotics to cover Gram-positive infections include vancomycin and to cover Gram-negative infections, i.e. a third-generation cephalosporin such as cefotaxime/ceftriaxone or ceftazidime (provides cover against *Pseudomonas aeruginosa*), or an aminoglycoside (e.g. gentamicin), should be given intraperitoneally.

23.4 Why is intraperitoneal dosing usually preferred to intravenous dosing?

Intraperitoneal dosing results in very high local concentrations of antibiotics, as achievement of the equivalent levels would require high and potentially toxic systemic doses. Also, peritoneal dosing can be given continuously or once daily in the case of intermittent dosing, when there should be a dwell time of at least 6 hours. Intraperitoneal dosing precludes the need for intravenous access and the possibility of subsequent intravascular catheter-related bloodstream infection. However, intravenous antibiotics may be indicated if there is believed to be associated systemic sepsis such as peritonitis associated with a perforated viscus.

Case history continued

The patient is started on intraperitoneal vancomycin and ceftazidime. *Pseudomonas aeruginosa* is isolated from the CAPD fluid.

Questions

23.5 Does the isolation of *Ps. aeruginosa* alter the antibiotic management?

23.6 Should the peritoneal dialysis catheter be removed?

Answers

23.5 Does the isolation of *Ps. aeruginosa* alter the antibiotic management?

Yes. As no Gram-positive organisms have been isolated, vancomycin can be discontinued and for *P. aeruginosa*, unlike for other Gram-negative infections, oral fluoroquinolones are recommended with or without concomitant intraperitoneal anti-pseudomonal antibiotics for approximately 21 days.

23.6 Should the peritoneal dialysis catheter be removed?

Yes, usually. Catheter removal is usually required for pseudomonas infection, where there is evidence of exit-site infection as evidenced by purulent drainage from the exit site (Fig. 23.1), or if there is recurrent infection.

Case history continued

The patient subsequently responds to treatment and returns to the CAPD programme. However, 2 years later, he develops another episode of peritonitis. Culture of the CAPD fluid is negative and he was not recently on antibiotics.

Questions

23.7 What might be the reason for culture-negative CAPD-related peritonitis?

23.8 How common is fungal peritonitis?

23.9 What key measures should be introduced in a CAPD programme to minimize dialysis-related infections?

23.10 Should patients on peritoneal dialysis receive antibiotic prophylaxis before lower gastrointestinal endoscopy?

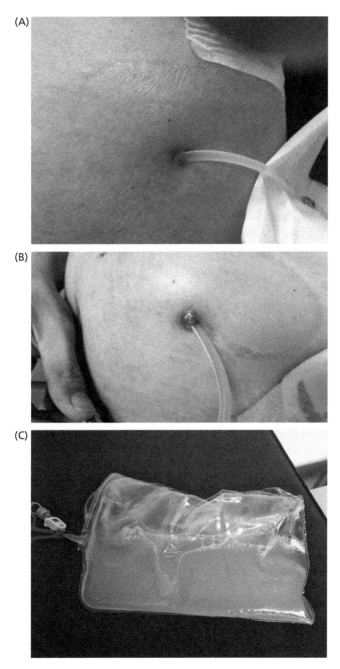

Figure 23.1 CAPD catheter exit site and peritonitis. (A) normal exit site; (B) infected exit site; (C) cloudy bag (see colour plate).

Reproduced courtesy of Annette Butler, Beaumont Hospital, Dublin, Ireland.

Answers

23.7 What might be the reason for culture-negative CAPD-related peritonitis?

This may be due to the administration of antibiotics when the CAPD sample is taken, fastidious or slow growing bacteria such as legionella, mycobacterial infection, or candida peritonitis.

23.8 How common is fungal peritonitis?

In most case series or surveillance studies of CAPD infection, fungi are responsible for less than 5% of total cases. The most common causes are *Candida albicans* and other *Candida* species. Catheter removal is required and an azole antifungal agent (e.g. fluconazole) or an echinocandin, especially if the isolate is not azole susceptible, is used for treatment.

23.9 What key measures should be introduced in a CAPD programme to minimize dialysis-related infections?

These can be categorized as specifically relating to dialysis and general measures. These are summarized in Table 23.1. Recent studies have not suggested that any particular catheter design is beneficial or that the location in the abdomen where the PD catheter is inserted is important in minimizing CAPD-related infection. Consequently, the emphasis is on personal hygiene, ongoing education, and training.

Table 23.1 Prevention of peritoneal dialysis-related infections

General measures	Specific measures	Not proven
Good standards of patient personal hygiene	Antibiotic prophylaxis before catheter insertion	Differences in catheter designs
Multi-disciplinary training on CAPD methodology	Eradication of nasal *S. aureus* carriage	Burying the catheter subcutaneously
Re-training and home visits	Y-set or twin bag system, preferred to 'spike' or luer lock device	Lateral abdominal catheter insertion
	Pre-procedural (e.g. endoscopy) antibiotic prophylaxis	Topical application of honey to catheter exit site

23.10 Should patients on peritoneal dialysis receive antibiotic prophylaxis before lower gastrointestinal endoscopy?

This is controversial and currently not routinely recommended. In theory, a lower gastrointestinal endoscopy procedure might lead to infection such as via a very small or unrecognized perforation but this is probably relatively uncommon. Therefore, it is probably best decided on a patient-by-patient basis and some guidelines recommend it.

Further reading

Ballinger AE, Palmer SC, Wiggins KJ, Nistori I, Craig GC, Strippoli GF, et al. Treatment for peritoneal dialysis-associated peritonitis (Review). *Cochrane Collaboration*. The Cochrane Library 2014.

Campbell DJ, Johnson DW, Mudge DW, Gallagher MP, Craig JC. Prevention of peritoneal dialysis-related infections. *Neph Dialysis Transplant* 2015; **30**: 1461–72.

Fried L, Bernardini J, Piraino B. Iatrogenic peritonitis: the need for prophylaxis. *Peritoneal Dialysis Internat* 2000; **20**: 343–5.

Li PK, Szeto CC, Piraino B , Bernardini J, Figueiredo AE, et al. ISPD Guidelines/ Recommendations. Peritoneal dialysis-related infections recommendations: 2010 update. *Peritoneal Dialysis Internat* 2010; **30**: 393–423.

Miles R, Hawley CM, McDonald SP, Brown FG, Rosman JB, et al. Predictors and outcomes of fungal peritonitis in peritoneal dialysis patients. *Kid Internat* 2009; **76**: 622–8.

Case 24

T H Nicholas Wong

Case history

A 43-year-old kidney transplant patient presents to clinic 9 months after transplantation. He is on tacrolimus and mycophenolate. His creatinine had been steadily increasing and there are concerns about rejection. Microscopy of a urine specimen is shown in Fig. 24.1.

Questions

24.1 What does the urine microscopy above show and what is the most likely cause of this finding?

24.2 What is the natural history, pathogenesis, and clinical features of this disease?

24.3 How is the diagnosis confirmed?

24.4 What are the screening options?

24.5 What are the treatment options?

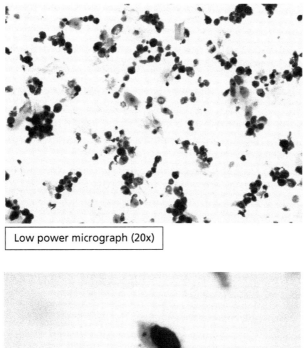

Low power micrograph (20x)

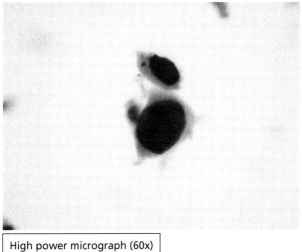

High power micrograph (60x)

Figure 24.1 Microscopy of urine (see colour plate).

Reproduced courtesy of Ian Roberts, Cellular Pathology, Oxford University Hospitals NHS Foundation Trust, Oxford, UK.

Answers

24.1 What does the urine microscopy above show and what is the most likely cause of this finding?

The low and high power micrographs show decoy cells. Decoy cells are infected epithelial cells with enlarged and abnormal nuclei and irregular shape that can sometimes mimic uroepithelial cancer cells. In the context of renal transplantation, immunosuppression and worsening creatinine function, this raises the possibility of BK virus-associated nephropathy (BKVAN).

Decoy cells may also be present in urine in John Cunningham/human polyomavirus 2 (JC) virus, cytomegalovirus (CMV), and adenovirus infections. Thus urine cytology with characteristic cytologic abnormalities is merely suggestive but not definitive for BKVAN with a positive predictive value of around 30% and a negative predictive value of 100%.

24.2 What is the natural history, pathogenesis, and clinical features of this disease?

BK virus is a human polyomavirus belonging to the *Polyomaviridae* family. The first BK virus was isolated from a urine specimen of a renal transplant patient with ureteric stenosis having the initials 'B.K.' Polyomaviruses are small (30–45 nm), non-enveloped viruses with a circular double-stranded DNA genome. BK virus can be transmitted via various routes including: faecal-oral, respiratory, through blood transfusions, organ transplantation, trans-placentally, and through seminal fluid.

Primary infection with BK virus is usually asymptomatic or associated with mild upper respiratory symptoms and 50% of children will have evidence of seroconversion by age 3 or 4. BK virus will then remain in a latent phase in the renal tubular epithelial cells (transitional epithelium, renal tubular epithelium, and parietal epithelium of Bowman's capsule). Around 80% of the population is infected with BK virus by adulthood.

The pathogenesis of reactivation disease involves a combination of factors, including host predisposition, target organ damage, and host immune function. Risk factors for reactivation include: BK virus seropositivity, older age, and high pre-transplant anti-BK virus IgG (immunoglobulin G).

Amongst renal transplant patients, BK virus causes tubule-interstitial nephritis and rarely ureteral stenosis. Haemorrhagic and non-haemorrhagic cystitis may occur with haemopoietic cell transplant recipients, but this is rarely seen in kidney transplant recipients. Other less common manifestations include pneumonitis, retinitis, liver disease, and meningoencephalitis.

Patients with BKVAN present with a slow rise in serum creatinine. This is usually asymptomatic and there are no clinical signs or symptoms of infection.

The prevalence of BKVAN ranges between 1% and 10% in renal transplant patients with the mean onset of disease around 44 weeks after transplant. Haemorrhagic cystitis occurs in approximately 10–25% of bone marrow transplant patients.

24.3 How is the diagnosis confirmed?

Renal biopsy remains the gold standard for confirming the diagnosis of BKVAN. Histologically, BKVAN is characterized by tubular atrophy and fibrosis with a lymphocytic infiltrate generally distinguished from rejection. The presence of intranuclear inclusion bodies staining positive for the large T antigen is pathognomonic for BKVAN. Correlation of histologic findings with BK viraemia is essential among patients with ambiguous histologic features.

Laboratory findings include an elevated creatinine, with either a normal urinalysis or evidence of pyuria, haematuria, or cellular casts consistent with interstitial nephritis. Serum antibodies against BK virus are not helpful in the diagnosis of BKVAN.

BKV infections progress through stages. Decoy cell appearance or BKV DNA is detected first in the urine, followed by DNA detection in the plasma (median of ~4 weeks), and then nephropathic changes in the kidney (median of ~12 weeks after BK viruria). Viruria and viraemia may be detected weeks to months before there is a detectable increase in the serum creatinine, suggesting that routine screening should be considered to prevent progression of asymptomatic BKV infection to clinically evident BKVAN.

BK plasma viral PCR is useful if negative (negative predictive value of 100%) for BKVAN and has a higher positive predictive value (between 50–60%) than that of decoy cells or BK viruria (see Table 24.1).

24.4 What are the screening options?

The optimal method of screening for BKVAN is unclear and recommendations vary. The American Society of Transplantation (AST) recommend screening of urine for

Table 24.1 Summary of BKV screening methods

Screening method	Positive predictive value (%)	Negative predictive value (%)	Sensitivity (%)	Specificity (%)
Decoy cells	29	100	25	84
BK urine PCR	40	100	100	78
BK plasma PCR	50-60	100	100	88

Adapted with permission from Sawinski D and Goral S (2015). BK virus infection: an update on diagnosis and treatment. *Nephrol Dial Transplant* 30(2):209–217. DOI: https://doi.org/10.1093/ndt/gfu023.

decoy cells or plasma for BKV viraemia, every 3 months for first 2 years, then annually until the fifth year post transplant. The Kidney Disease: Improving Global Outcomes (KDIGO) recommend screening via plasma BKV PCR monthly for the first 3–6 months, then every 3 months until the end of the first year post transplant. Studies have shown that BK viraemia, even without overt BKVAN, is associated with poorer graft function on long-term follow-up, suggesting that earlier intervention in the course of BKV infection (e.g. at the stage of viruria, before viraemia develops) may improve long-term graft outcomes.

24.5 What are the treatment options?

There is currently no specific antiviral for BK virus, and reducing immunosuppression remains the mainstay of treatment for BKVAN. Clearance of BK viraemia correlates with nephropathy resolution. Agents have been proposed to treat BKVAN, such as cidofovir, leflunomide, quinolones, and intravenous immunoglobulin (IVIG). In the case of cidofovir, there is evidence of its use for treating refractory BK nephropathy with stabilization of renal function. However, the mechanism of action for cidofovir in BKVAN is unclear, given that cidofovir inhibits viral DNA polymerase (e.g. for the treatment of CMV retinitis) but the BK virus genome does not encode a DNA polymerase. Leflunomide is a pyrimidine synthesis inhibitor which is widely used in the treatment of rheumatoid arthritis. In BK nephropathy, leflunomide inhibits mitochondrial enzymes involved in producing metabolites required for cell cycle progression, preventing expansion of activated lymphocytes. In a study of 17 patients, the use of both leflunomide and a reduction in immunosuppression resulted in viral clearance or a decrease in viraemia in 15 patients (88%). The proposed mechanism of action of quinolones is interference with large T antigen helicase activity for BK virus both *in vivo* and *in vitro*. Support for IVIG use in BK nephropathy is mixed.

Further reading

Ambalathingal GR, Francis RS, Smyth MJ, Smith C, Khanna R. BK polyomavirus: clinical aspects, immune regulation, and emerging therapies. *Clin Microbiol Rev* 2017; **30**: 503–28.

Barth H, Solis M, Lepiller Q, et al. 45 years after the discovery of human polyomaviruses BK and JC: Time to speed up the understanding of associated diseases and treatment approaches. *Crit Rev Microbiol* 2017; **43**: 178–95.

Lamarche C, Orio J, Collette S, Sueur C, Caillard S, et al. BK polyomavirus and the transplanted kidney: immunopathology and therapeutic approaches. *Transplantation* 2016; **100**: 2276–87.

Sawinski D, Goral S. BK virus infection: an update on diagnosis and treatment. *Nephrol Dial Transplant* 2014; **30**: 209–17.

Case 25

Andrew Woodhouse

Case history

A 23-year-old man is referred to Infectious Diseases by the acute medical team with 4 days of fever and occasional cough 5 weeks after returning from a 3-month trip to Africa. He took daily doxycycline as malaria prophylaxis and was well throughout his trip. He spent time in Kenya, Uganda, and Malawi and took part in a number of water-based recreational activities including rafting and a lake-based diving course. He recalls development of an itchy rash on his legs and arms at one stage after a single day diving.

There are no abnormalities on clinical examination. Chest X-ray (CXR) shows a poorly defined infiltrate in the right mid-zone and blood tests show an eosinophil count of 2.5×10^9/L (normal range 0.05–0.5×10^9/L) but no other significant abnormalities. He has been started on penicillin and clarithromycin for possible pneumonia in the Emergency Department (ED) and a malaria antigen test is negative as are two malaria smears.

Questions

25.1 Why is schistosomiasis a consideration in this case?

25.2 What stage of schistosomiasis infection might he now be presenting with?

25.3 How can the diagnosis of schistosomiasis be confirmed?

25.4 If acute schistosomiasis is suspected should treatment be commenced?

Answers

25.1 Why is schistosomiasis a consideration in this case?

He has been at risk of acquiring schistosomiasis based on his freshwater exposure in sub-Saharan Africa. His history of an itchy rash after diving might represent 'swimmers itch'—an urticarial response to schistosome cerceriae penetrating the skin at the time of infection.

25.2 What stage of schistosomiasis infection might he now be presenting with?

Based on his history, symptoms, and peripheral eosinophilia, this could be a presentation of acute schistosomiasis (AS), also known eponymously as 'Katayama fever'. Clinical features of AS include fever, myalgia, urticarial rash, dyspnoea, and generalized systemic symptoms. The incubation period varies from between 3 and 12 weeks from exposure although the majority of primary infections are asymptomatic. Full blood count typically shows peripheral eosinophilia. The clinical syndrome is a result of the host's hypersensitivity response to migrating schistosomes and early egg production. Pulmonary symptoms may be associated with an infiltrate on chest X-ray (CXR). Rare cases of neurological involvement have been described in early illness including involvement of the spinal cord causing a transverse myelitis but this can occur without other manifestations of AS and is probably due to mistaken migration of adult worms into the brain or spinal cord with a consequent local inflammatory response.

25.3 How can the diagnosis of schistosomiasis be confirmed?

The diagnosis of schistosomiasis depends on the stage of infection and parasite burden. Detection of schistosome ova by microscopy in concentrated stool or urine samples remains the gold standard of diagnosis in established infection (Fig 25.1). In early, symptomatic acute infection it may be difficult to detect ova in stool or urine as egg production and deposition may be initially light. Serology can be helpful, particularly in travellers who are unlikely to have pre-existing antibodies. Detection of antibody by enzyme-linked immunosorbent assay (ELISA) or indirect haemagglutination assay (IHA) has a high sensitivity and seroconversion with detectable IgM antibody can occur as early as 4 weeks after infection. Initial negative serology does not exclude the diagnosis in early infection. Newer techniques, including antigen detection and PCR to detect the parasite, have been developed but are not widely available and await confirmation of their role in diagnosis of acute and chronic infection.

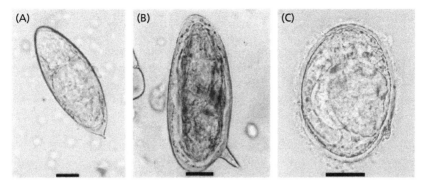

Figure 25.1 Schistosomiasis eggs. (A) *S. haematobium* (in urine); (B) *S. mansoni* (in stool); (C) *S. japonicum* (in stool). [Scale: bar = 25 μ m] (see colour plate).

Reproduced with permission from World Health Organization. (1994). *Bench Aids for the Diagnosis of Faecal Parasites*. Geneva, Switzerland: World Health Organization.

Histology is unlikely to be helpful in AS but examination of rectal 'snip' biopsies or biopsies of bladder lesions increase diagnostic sensitivity in chronically infected cases where egg excretion in urine or faeces may have reduced.

25.4 If acute schistosomiasis is suspected should treatment be commenced?

Not necessarily. The main treatment in AS is symptomatic and most cases will settle spontaneously over a number of weeks. There is little evidence for any specific treatment intervention and experts vary in their opinion. Anti-inflammatory strategies are thought to be indicated including with corticosteroids if symptoms are severe. Praziquantel is the drug treatment of choice for schistosomiasis but may be less effective in early infection when worms are immature and if used acutely there is a risk of exacerbating the inflammatory response hence recommendations to use adjunctive steroids. Waiting for the acute illness to subside before using praziquantel or re-treating after a few months may improve the likelihood of eradicating infection.

Case history continued

A travelling companion of the patient described presents 12 months after returning from Africa worried that he may have schistosomiasis. He has noticed occasional what he thinks is blood in his urine. He also spent time on a diving course.

Questions

25.5 How should he be investigated?

25.6 If he presented with intermittent abdominal pain and eosinophilia what other investigations might be required?

25.7 What is the treatment for schistosomiasis?

Answers

25.5 How should he be investigated?

He may have urinary tract schistosomiasis, most likely caused by S. *haematobium* (Figure 25.1). He should have haematuria confirmed and midday urines examined for ova. Schistosoma serology should be requested and a full blood count to look for eosinophilia. A renal tract ultrasound and cystoscopy should be considered, particularly if ova are not detected on microscopy. Biopsy of inflammatory lesions in the bladder may show granulomas and schistosome eggs (Fig. 25.2).

25.6 If he presented with intermittent abdominal pain and eosinophilia what other investigations might be required?

Gastrointestinal schistosomiasis can manifest as abdominal pain, intermittent diarrhoea, and occasionally with rectal bleeding. S. *mansoni* and S. *intercalatum* are the common species causing gastrointestinal disease. Stool samples for

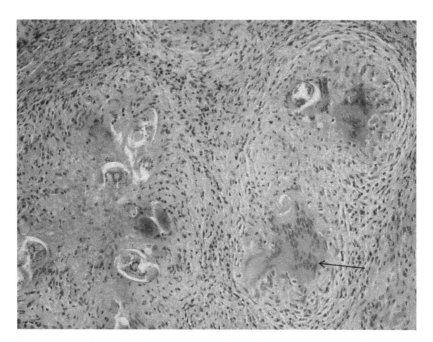

Figure 25.2 Multiple schistosoma ova associated with a granulomatous inflammatory response, including multinucleated giant cells (arrow). H&E, ×200 (see colour plate).

Reproduced courtesy of University Hospitals Birmingham NHS Foundation Trust, UK.

microscopy looking for ova are required. Concentration techniques improve the yield. Abdominal ultrasound may show a characteristic pattern of widening of the periportal spaces progressing to periportal fibrosis (Symmer's pipe-stem fibrosis). Hepatocellular function is preserved and treatment can result in regression of the early changes.

25.7 What is the treatment for schistosomiasis?

The treatment of choice is praziquantal for all species of schistosomes. The mechanism of action of praziquantal is incompletely understood but it is active against adult worms. For *S. mansoni* and *S. haematobium* a dose of 40 mg/kg (as a single or 2 divided doses) is recommended, with a dose of 60 mg/kg (as 2 divided doses) for *S. japonicum* and *S. mekongi*. The artemesinin derivatives used to treat malaria show activity against less mature larval forms of the parasite and combination therapy with praziquantal may have potential.

Further reading

Clernix, J, Van Gompel A. Schistosomiasis in travellers and migrants. *Travel Med Infect Dis* 2011; **9**: 6–24.

Colley DG, Bustinday AL, Secor WE, King CH. Human schistosomiasis. *Lancet* 2014; **383**: 2253–64.

Ferrari TCA, Moreira PRR. Neuroschistosomiasis: clinical symptoms and pathogenesis. *Lancet Neurol* 2011; **10**: 853–64.

Ross AG, Vickers D, Olds GR, Shah SM, McManus DP. Katayama syndrome. *Lancet Infect Dis* 2007; 7: 218–24.

Central nervous system infections

Case 26 – Case 30

Case 26

Hilary Humphreys

Case history

A 72-year-old man is admitted via the Emergency Department (ED) with a fever, headache, and confusion. There is a background history of diabetes mellitus and chronic obstructive pulmonary disease. On examination, he has a temperature of 39.5 °C, his blood pressure is normal but there is some neck stiffness. There is no skin rash and both the Brudzinski and Kernig signs are negative.

Questions

26.1 Does the absence of both Brudzinski and Kernig signs exclude the diagnosis of meningitis?

26.2 Should this patient have cranial imaging before a lumbar puncture (LP) is performed?

26.3 What key laboratory techniques are important in confirming a diagnosis of bacterial meningitis?

Answers

26.1 Does the absence of both Brudzinski and Kernig signs exclude the diagnosis of meningitis?

No. In adults, the most common clinical manifestations of bacterial meningitis are fever, headache, neck stiffness, and altered mental status. Other clinical signs have a low sensitivity and their absence does not exclude the diagnosis.

26.2 Should this patient have cranial imaging before a lumbar puncture (LP) is performed?

No. Cranial imaging is however recommended before an LP for patients with focal neurological deficits, continuous or uncontrolled seizures, a Glasgow Coma Scale of 12 or less, and in severely immunocompromised patients (Fig. 26.1).

26.3 What key laboratory techniques are important in confirming a diagnosis of bacterial meningitis?

Cerebrospinal fluid (CSF) leucocyte count and differential CSF glucose compared to blood glucose and total CSF protein, as well as microscopy and culture are base-line tests. In addition, blood cultures should be taken and both blood and CSF should be analysed by polymerase chain reaction (PCR) to detect common causes, such as

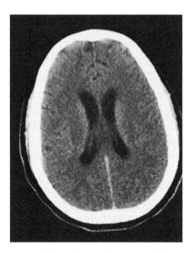

Figure 26.1 CT scan showing obliteration of the sulci, with moderate hydrocephalus, including of the temporal horns of the lateral ventricles, a contra-indication to an LP.
Reproduced courtesy of Seamus Looby, Beaumont Hospital, Dublin, Ireland.

Streptococcus pneumoniae and *Neisseria meningitidis*. A high proportion of patients with pneumococcal meningitis have positive blood cultures. Other tests that may or may not be available locally include CSF lactate and latex agglutination of CSF to detect bacterial antigens.

Case history continued

The patient is started on antibiotics and corticosteroids. An LP is performed. The CSF has a white cell count of 450 × 10⁶L with 90% polymorphs (normal, < 5 lymphocytes, no polymorphs), a protein of 1500 mg/L (normal < 430 mg/L), and a CSF glucose level which is less than 1 mmol/L; the blood glucose is 4.5 mmol/L (the normal CSF glucose is ≥ 2/3 of blood glucose). Microscopy reveals the presence of Gram-positive diplococci. Culture and PCR of CSF and blood are all positive for *Streptococcus pneumoniae*. Susceptibility test results indicate that the isolate has a minimum inhibitory concentration (MIC) of 0.06 mg/ ml to benzylpenicillin.

Questions

26.4 What empirical antibiotic treatment should this patient have been started on and what changes would be made based on the MIC result above?

26.5 What are the risk factors for non-susceptibility/resistance to benzylpenicillin amongst pneumococci?

26.6 Why are corticosteroids given with antibiotics for the treatment of bacterial meningitis? What effect do they have?

26.7 Should the pneumococcal isolate be sent for serotyping?

26.8 Should this patient be vaccinated to prevent further episodes of invasive pneumococcal disease?

26.9 Which vaccine should this patient receive if not previously vaccinated?

Answers

26.4 What empirical antibiotic treatment should this patient have been started on and what changes would be made based on the MIC result above?

Current recommendations for empirical antibiotics in this age group are a third-generation cephalosporin such as cefotaxime or ceftriaxone. If the patient comes from a country where penicillin resistance amongst pneumococci is common, vancomycin should also be added. In patients over 60 or who are immuncompromised, high-dose intravenous (IV) amoxicillin should be added to cover *Listeria monocytogenes*. This patient is in this age group and also has diabetes mellitus so should receive empiric Listeria treatment. When the MIC is available, if the isolate is penicillin-susceptible, the third-generation cephalosporin should subsequently be changed to high-dose benzylpenicillin (Table 26.1). Other antibiotics may be discontinued as the patient has a penicillin-susceptible pneumococcus as the sole cause of meningitis.

26.5 What are the risk factors for non-susceptibility/resistance to benzylpenicillin amongst pneumococci?

The proportion of isolates causing invasive pneumococcal disease (IPD) that are penicillin non-susceptible varies from over 40% in some countries to less than 10%

Table 26.1 Antibiotic treatment and duration for specific causes of community-acquired meningitis

Microbe	Antibiotic(s)	Duration
Streptococcus pneumoniae		
penicillin-susceptible	benzylpenicillin	10–14 days
penicillin-resistant	cefotaxime/ceftriaxone	10–14 days
cephalosporin-resistant	vancomycin + rifampicin or linezolid	10–14 days
Neisseria meningitidis	benzylpenicillin	5–7 days
Haemophilus influenza		
amoxicillin/ampicillin susceptible	amoxicillin/ampicillin	7–10 days
amoxicillin/ampicillin-resistant	cefotaxime/ceftriaxone	7–10 days
Listeria monocytogenes	amoxicillin/ampicillin/benzylpenicillin	≥ 21 days
	+/– gentamicin	

in the United Kingdom. The risk factors include recent antibiotic use, hospitalization, attending day care, infection caused by certain serotypes, and immunosuppression.

26.6 Why are corticosteroids given with antibiotics for the treatment of bacterial meningitis? What effect do they have?

Corticosteroids are believed to reduce inflammation associated with bacterial meningitis. They should be given with the first doses of antibiotics or very shortly afterwards.

Corticosteroids result in a small reduction in mortality due to infection with *S. pneumoniae* and less severe hearing loss in children due to *H. influenza*. Generally, corticosteroid treatment is safe but may be associated with recurrent fever.

26.7 Should the pneumococcal isolate be sent for serotyping?

Yes. Serotyping helps identify the common pattern of strains causing IPD and whether or not these are covered by current vaccination schedules. Also, some serotypes are associated with particular infections. For example, serotypes 1, 3, 5, 7F, 8, and 19A are associated with empyema and 3, 6A, 6B, and 6C are associated with meningitis.

26.8 Should this patient be vaccinated to prevent further episodes of invasive pneumococcal disease?

Yes, if the patient has not been vaccinated in the last 5 years. Patients over 65 years of age and with a chronic illness—diabetes mellitus and chronic obstructive pulmonary disease—should be routinely vaccinated.

26.9 Which vaccine should this patient receive if not previously vaccinated?

Hitherto, the recommendation has been to administer a single dose of the pneumococcal polysaccharide vaccine which protects against 23 serotypes (PPV23). It is recommended in the United Kingdom that this vaccination be repeated at 5-year intervals for patients with asplenia and chronic kidney disease. However, the recent introduction for children of pneumococcal conjugate vaccines, such as PCV 13 which covers 13 common serotypes and which also results in a T-cell response, has altered the epidemiology of IPD. There has been a reduction in IPD amongst children and in other age groups, including the elderly. There is now a view that there may be a case for adults receiving PCV13 as well as PPV23 as this results in greater opsonophagocytic activity with potentially better protection. Also, the combination of PPV23 and PCV13 theoretically cover up to 78% of all potential infections. Further studies are likely to clarify the relationship between the two vaccines and lead to more definitive guidelines on when and in what order the combination of vaccines should be used.

Further reading

Brouwer MC, McIntyre P, Prasad K, van de Beek D. Corticosteroids for acute bacterial meningitis. *Cochrane Data Syst Rev* 2013; 6: CD00405. doi: 10.1002/14651858.CD004405.pub4.

Falkenhorst G, Remschmidt C, Harder T, Hummers-Pradier E, Wichmann O, et al. Effectiveness of the 23-valent pneumococcal polysaccharide vaccine (PPV23) against pneumococcal disease in the elderly: systematic review and meta-analysis. *PLoS One* 2017; **12**: e0169368. doi:10.1371/journal.

Grabenstein JD, Musey LK. Differences in serious clinical outcomes of infection caused by specific pneumococcal serotypes among adults. *Vaccine* 2014; **32**: 2399–405.

Kim L, McGee L, Tomcyzk S, Beall B. Biological and epidemiological features of antibiotic-resistant *Streptococcus pneumoniae* in pre- and post- conjugate vaccine eras: a United States perspective. *Clin Microbiol Rev* 2016; **29**: 525–52.

McGill F, Heyderman RS, Michael BD, Defres S, Beeching NJ, et al. The UK joint specialist societies guideline on the diagnosis and management of acute meningitis and meningococcal sepsis in immunocompetent adults. *J Infect* 2016; **72**: 405–38.

Case 27

Hilary Humphreys

Case history

A 45-year-old female presents to the Emergency Department (ED) with a 5-day history of malaise, fatigue, and feeling feverish. In the last 24 hours, she has been described as acting strangely and has just had a seizure. On examination, she has a temperature of 38 °C but has no localizing neurological signs. She is disorientated in time and space, with a Glasgow Coma Scale (GCS) of 13, but the physical examination is otherwise normal.

Questions

27.1 What is the differential diagnosis?

27.2 What is the most likely microbial cause?

27.3 How does the aetiology differ in the immunocompromised host?

Answers

27.1 What is the differential diagnosis?

The presence of fever, a seizure and altered behaviour over a relatively short period are suggestive of encephalitis. However, the initial presentation could indicate a space-occupying lesion such as a tumour and a cerebral vascular event is also possible. Imaging with either a contrast computerized tomography (CT) or magnetic resonance imaging (MRI) would confirm or exclude both (Figures 27.1 and 27.2).

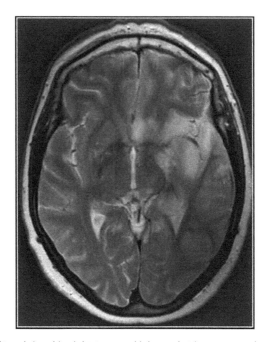

Figure 27.1 Altered signal in right temporal lobe and striatum strongly suggestive of HSV encephalitis.

Reproduced courtesy of Michael Farrell, Neuropathologist, Beaumont Hospital, Dublin, Ireland.

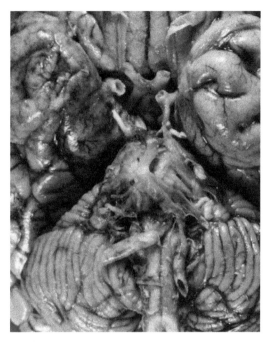

Figure 27.2 Bilaterial haemorrhagic temporal lobe necrosis on post-mortem of a patient that died of HSV encephalitis (see colour plate).

Reproduced courtesy of Michael Farrell, Neuropathologist, Beaumont Hospital, Dublin, Ireland.

27.2 What is the most likely microbial cause?

Herpes simplex virus (HSV) accounts for approximately 40–50% of cases of sporadic encephalitis where a cause is determined, HSV 1 being responsible for most of these. Although viruses are the most common cause of encephalitis, a specific aetiology is found in only about half of all cases, notwithstanding advances in diagnostic techniques. Other viral causes in the immunocompetent host include varicella-zoster, influenza, mumps, and measles in an unvaccinated individual, and enteroviruses, although these viruses are more commonly associated with aseptic meningitis. A travel history is essential (e.g. to suspect West Nile virus), and worldwide, rabies is the commonest cause of encephalitis. There are many arboviruses such as West Nile virus, Japanese encephalitis virus, tick-borne encephalitis viruses, and Nipah and Hendra viruses which have specific geographical distributions. Consequently, a travel history should routinely be taken to determine if these need to investigated for.

27.3 How does the aetiology differ in the immunocompromised host?

In addition to the causes listed above, a number of other agents should be considered, particularly other herpesviruses such as cytomegalovirus, Epstein–Barr virus and human herpes virus type 6. HIV infection may also be associated with an encephalopathy. Free-living amoeba—for example, *Balamuthia mandrillaris*, which has a global distribution especially in fresh water—has a high case-fatality rate of more than 90%. Details of some of these agents are presented in Table 27.1.

Table 27.1 Features of some less common or opportunist causes of encephalitis

Pathogen	Epidemiology	Diagnosis	Management	Other
Human herpes virus-6 (HHV-6)	90% of adults infected during childhood and reactivates, especially in stem cell transplant patients	HHV-6 DNA detected by PCR	Ganciclovir, foscarnet, or both	Blood serology is not predictive
Rabies virus	Worldwide with few exceptions	Saliva, skin biopsies, serum and CSF for PCR and immunofluorescence	Largely supportive care, e.g. ventilation. Rabies vaccine and rabies immunoglobulin should be administered	Mortality approaches 100%. Vaccinate those at risk, e.g. veterinarians
West Nile virus	More common in parts of Europe and United States, mosquito-transmitted. Now endemic in the United States.	CSF-IgM but PCR may be necessary if poor humoral response	Supportive care only	Mortality of 25%, highest in the elderly
Balamuthia Mandrillaris	Ubiquitous in soil and fresh water. Greater risk in hotter climates. Depleted CD4+ T-cells a risk	Non-validated molecular methods	Experimental treatment with albendazole, fluconazole, and other agents	Severe illness with 90% mortality

CSF, cerebrospinal fluid; PCR, polymerase chain reaction.

Case history continued

The patient is admitted to hospital and routine blood tests are normal. However, cerebral imaging shows altered signals due to oedema in the right temporal lobe strongly suggestive of HSV encephalitis (Fig. 27.1 and Fig. 27.2). A lumbar puncture is performed and in the CSF, there is pleoycytosis, with a white cell count of 150×10^6/L, 90% lymphocytes (normal < 5). The protein is slightly elevated but the CSF glucose is within normal limits compared to serum glucose.

Questions

27.4 What approaches are taken to confirm a laboratory diagnosis of encephalitis?

27.5 What is the likely outcome in this patient and in other patients with encephalitis?

27.6 What non-infectious cause of encephalitis may mimic infection?

27.7 What are the principles of the management of viral encephalitis?

Answers

27.4 What approaches are taken to confirm a laboratory diagnosis of encephalitis?

As most cases of encephalitis are viral in aetiology, there is increasing reliance on molecular methods including monoplex PCR assays, multiplex assays, and, more recently, metagenomics. Antibody analysis of CSF is still used to detect immunoglobulin M (IgM) in CSF to confirm a diagnosis of West Nile virus and for the diagnosis of neurosyphilis but otherwise, serology is not helpful. High-throughput RNA sequencing performed on brain biopsies and CSF in recent years has identified astrovirus as a cause of encephalitis. Therefore it is possible that in the future other previously unrecognized causes of encephalitis may be identified. However, neuroimaging, ideally MR but otherwise contrast CT, is essential; focal lesions as opposed to diffuse changes strongly suggest HSV.

27.5 What is the likely outcome in this patient and in other patients with encephalitis?

With the early administration of appropriate antiviral treatment, the mortality from HSV encephalitis has fallen to less than 10%. However, a significant proportion of survivors have functional and cognitive impairment. West Nile virus encephalitis has a mortality rate of about 20% which is worse in the elderly and those presenting with coma or cranial nerve deficit. Encephalitis due to rabies virus is almost always fatal with few exceptions.

27.6 What non-infectious cause of encephalitis may mimic infection?

Auto-immune forms of encephalitis are increasingly recognised and diagnosed in patients where tests for an infectious cause are negative. These forms of encephalitis are often associated with rigidity and myoclonus. Autoimmune encephalitis may be divided into several groups of diseases: those with pathogenic antibodies to cell surface proteins; those with antibodies to intracellular synaptic proteins; T-cell diseases associated with antibodies to intracellular antigens; and those associated with other autoimmune disorders. Many forms of autoimmune encephalitis are paraneoplastic and each of these conveys a distinct risk profile for various tumours. Rarely, and somewhat paradoxically, aciclovir toxicity may manifest with symptoms of confusion and convulsions. Measurement of plasma levels may assist in making this diagnosis.

27.7 What are the principles of the management of viral encephalitis?

High-dose aciclovir—for example, 10 mg/kg, administered intravenously every 8 hours for 21 days—is recommended for HSV encephalitis and this is associated with reduced morbidity and mortality. Therapy must be initiated empirically as soon as a diagnosis of encephalitis is suspected—if subsequent investigations reveal a different aetiology, the aciclovir can be stopped. Aciclovir is also recommended for varicella-zoster virus but there are no clinical trials to support this. There are no recommended treatments for other causes of viral encephalitis although foscarnet has been used against human herpes virus (HHV) 6.

Corticosteroids are used to treat auto-immune causes of encephalitis and it has been suggested that steroids should also be used with acyclovir for HSV encephalitis to reduce vasogenic oedema and any mass effect. Monitoring of intra-cranial pressure to minimize the consequences of cerebral oedema, ventilation for patients seriously obtunded, and the early and effective treatment of seizures, usually in the intensive care unit, are also all important supportive measures.

Further Reading

He T, Kaplan S, Kamboj M, Tang Y-W. Laboratory diagnosis of central nervous system infection. *Curr Infect Dis Rep* 2016; 18–35. doi:10.1007/s11908-016-0545-6.

Kennedy PGE, Quan P-L, Lipkin WI. Viral encephalitis of unknown cause: current perspective and recent advances. *Viruses* 2017; **9**: 138. doi: 10.3390/v9060138.

Saylor D, Thakur K, Venkatesan A. Acute encephalitis in the immunocompromised individual. *Curr Opin Infect Dis* 2015; **28**: 330–6.

Solomon T, Michael BD, Smith PE, et al. National encephalitis guidelines development and stakeholder groups. management of suspected viral encephalitis in adults--Association of British Neurologists and British Infection Association National Guidelines. *J Infect* 2012; **64**: 347–73.

Tyler KL. Acute viral encephalitis. *N Engl J Med* 2018; **379**: 557–66.

Case 28

Hilary Humphreys

Case history

A 47-year-old tax consultant presents to the Emergency Department (ED) with a 3–4 week history of headache, fever, and altered behaviour. His partner has noticed that he has become forgetful of late and irritable. Three hours previously, he had a seizure. He has a background history of acute myeloid leukaemia for which he has been on chemotherapy and steroids in the past 3 months. He lives in the countryside and one of his hobbies is to keep ornamental fish in a pond. He received co-amoxiclav 5 days earlier prescribed by his General Practitioner (GP) who had diagnosed sinusitis. On examination, he has a temperature of 38.5 °C and a heart rate of 120 beats per minute but his blood pressure and respiratory rate are normal. He has no papilloedema and no localizing neurological signs. He undergoes an MRI, which shows an irregular peripheral-enhancing lesion in the right anterior temporal lobe with surrounding oedema thought possibly to represent a metastatic deposit, a primary tumour, or, most likely, an abscess (Fig. 28.1).

Questions

28.1 What initial investigations should this patient undergo?

28.2 What would be the next appropriate step in the management of this presumed abscess?

28.3 What laboratory techniques are available to confirm a microbiological diagnosis?

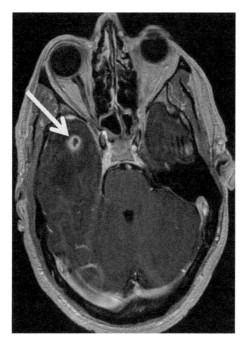

Figure 28.1 MRI showing abscess in the right anterior temporal lobe (arrow).

Answers

28.1 What initial investigations should this patient undergo?

In addition to routine bloods, such as white cell count and C-reactive protein (CRP), blood cultures should be taken as he is pyrexial, and a lumbar puncture (LP) considered but not until after a computerized tomography (CT) scan or MRI excludes raised intracranial pressure due to a space-occupying lesion (see Case 26).

28.2 What would be the next appropriate step in the management of this presumed abscess?

Historically, a brain abscess was managed by open drainage via a craniotomy. However, with more sophisticated imaging techniques, abscesses are increasingly managed via stereotactic aspiration under radiological guidance or via a burr hole. Both of these are less invasive and associated with a better outcome. However, the feasibility of stereotactic aspiration depends on the location and the size of the abscess. It may not be possible to aspirate multiple abscesses or those less than 1 cm in diameter. While stereotactic aspiration may provide a microbiological diagnosis it may not result in effective source control, complete or near-complete drainage of pus. Therefore repeat aspiration or an open craniotomy is sometimes required, especially for large abscesses > 3 cm in diameter.

28.3 What laboratory techniques are available to confirm a microbiological diagnosis?

Most brain abscesses are due to pyogenic bacteria, for example, those in the *Streptococcus milleri* group (*Streptococcus intermedius, anginosus*, and *constellatus*). These are often seen on Gram stain, and can usually be cultured, unless the patient is on antibiotics. It is increasingly recognized that polymicrobial infection can occur, and in patients with underlying immune deficiency as here, more fastidious organisms or opportunist pathogens may be the cause. Hence, conventional cultures may be negative even in the absence of current or recent antibiotics. In addition to Gram stain, direct and enrichment culture and prolonged anaerobic incubation, molecular methods are increasingly used. These include PCR amplification of the 16S rDNA gene, followed by cloning and sequencing. This has resulted in the detection of multiple pathogens in brain abscesses not detected by culture and organisms not previously recognized as causing brain abscesses such as *Mycoplasma* spp. Additionally, this technique is useful in patients on antibiotics or who have recently being treated as in the case here (co-amoxiclav by his GP), and where cultures are sterile. Other molecular techniques used to identify or further characterize/ type organisms include randomly amplified polymorphic DNA PCR (RAPD) and multilocus sequence typing (MLST).

Case history continued

The patient undergoes a stereotactic aspiration procedure which results in the collection of 1.5 ml of pus. Inflammatory cells are seen on Gram stain (but no organisms). There is no growth after prolonged incubation. Histology indicates an abscess with a fibrous wall (Fig. 28.2) and special stains for possible microbes are negative. He is commenced empirically on anti-infective therapy. Shortly afterwards, a report from the reference laboratory indicates that the 16S rDNA gene amplification analysis is positive for *Nocardia* spp.

Questions

28.4 What anti-infective treatment would you initially recommend for this patient?

28.5 How may this patient have acquired *Nocardia* spp.?

28.6 How should this patient be specifically treated for *Nocardia* spp.?

28.7 For how long should this patient be treated?

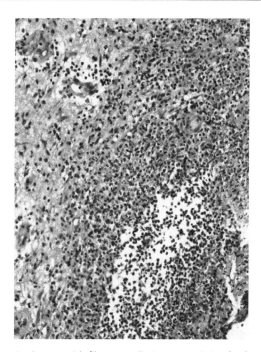

Figure 28.2 Chronic abscess with fibrous wall. Grocott staining for fungi was negative (see colour plate).

Reproduced courtesy of Michael Farrell, Neuropathologist, Beaumont Hospital, Dublin, Ireland.

Answers

28.4 What anti-infective treatment would you initially recommend for this patient?

Most guidelines recommend as empirical treatment for a brain abscess a third-generation cephalosporin or a carbapenem because of the broad spectrum of cover and good penetration into the brain, with an anaerobic agent such as metronidazole. In the patient described with a background of immunosuppression, there is a case to be made for adding to this, and from the start, an antifungal agent such as lipososmal amphotericin B or voriconazole.

28.5 How may this patient have acquired *Nocardia* spp.?

Nocardia are aerobic filamentous Gram-positive branching rods and part of the normal human flora. They are also found in soil and in water environments which may be relevant in the case of this patient given his hobby of keeping ornamental fish. Eighty species of *Nocardia* have been identified but those belonging to *N. asteroides* complex are most commonly associated with human disease, which can affect most organs. While this infection can occur in immunocompetent patients, most cases occur in those with some underlying immune deficiency, especially involving T-cell function, especially high-dose prolonged glucocorticoid therapy, malignancy, organ transplantation, and HIV infection. If associated with HIV infection or other immunosuppressed states, other possible sites should be sought such as the respiratory tract and the skin (often associated with disseminated infection).

28.6 How should this patient be specifically treated for *Nocardia* spp.?

There are no randomized controlled trials to guide optimum antimicrobial treatment. Isolates of *Nocardia* spp. are variably resistant to antibiotics but most experts agree that trimethoprim-sulfamethoxazole is the initial empiric drug of choice (with or without a carbapenem), and most isolates are susceptible. Susceptibility testing should be carried out if an isolate is cultured in case there is resistance or the patient cannot tolerate trimethoprim-sulfamethoxazole. Alternative agents include amikacin, imipenem, and extended-spectrum fluroquinolones such as moxifloxacin.

28.7 For how long should this patient be treated?

It is not clear how long patients with central nervous system infection due to *Nocardia* spp. should be treated. Prolonged therapy—6–12 months—is usually recommended and where there is immunosuppression, treatment for at least a year is preferred.

Further reading

Kennedy KJ, Chung KH, Bowden FJ, Mews PJ, Pik JH, et al. A cluster of nocardial brain abscesses. *Surg Neurol* 2007; **68**: 43–9.

Mishra AK, Dufour H, Roche P-H, Lonjon M, Raoult D, et al. Molecular revolution in the diagnosis of microbial brain abscesses. *Eur J Clin Microbiol Infect Dis* 2014; **33**: 2083–93.

Mootsikapun P, Intarapoka B, Liawnoraset W. Nocardiosis in Srinagarind Hospital, Thailand: review of 70 cases from 1996–2001. *Int J Infect Dis* 2005; **9**: 154–8.

Ratnaike TE, Das S, Gregson BA, Mendelow AD. A review of brain abscess surgical treatment – 78 years: aspiration versus excision. *World Neurosurg* 2011; **76**: 431–6.

Sonneville R, Ruimy R, Benzonana N, Riffaud L, Carsin A, et al. An update on bacterial brain abscess in immunocompetent patients. *Clin Microbiol Infect* 2017; **23**: 614–20.

Case 29

Lucinda Barrett and Bridget L. Atkins

Case history

An 18-year-old man presents with a decreased level of consciousness after a few weeks' history of headache and vomiting. Brain imaging demonstrates a mass lesion in the pineal gland with associated haemorrhage and hydrocephalus. He undergoes urgent neurosurgery for evacuation of blood, lesion biopsy, and the insertion of an extra-ventricular drain (EVD). Post-operatively he is admitted to the neurosurgical intensive care unit (NICU) where he remains intubated to optimize management of raised intracranial pressure (ICP). On day 3 he becomes febrile.

Questions

29.1 What are the possible causes of his fever?

29.2 What investigations should be requested?

Answers

29.1 What are the possible causes of his fever?

Fever in this scenario may be due to infection, a post-operative inflammatory response, or driven by the central nervous system in the context of brain tumour, bleeding, and surgery. If his haemodynamic state is one of hypotension and tachycardia, infection is more likely. The differential is wide in an NICU patient. Chest, vascular line, and urinary catheter-associated infection are all possibilities. In addition, his EVD and cranial surgical site are other potential sources.

29.2 What investigations should be requested?

Following full clinical examination, he should have a full septic screen including blood cultures (both peripheral and through any long lines), urine, and lower respiratory samples such as a broncho-alveolar lavage (BAL) for quantitative culture. Cerebrospinal fluid (CSF) should be sampled, using immaculate aseptic technique, from the EVD for cell count, Gram stain, culture, protein, and glucose. He should have a chest radiograph, and repeat brain imaging should be considered if there is any change in his neurological status.

Case history continued

The following results are obtained from CSF sampled from the EVD: white blood cell count (WCC) 320 cells/µl, with polymorphs (P) 200 and lymphocytes (L) 120, and red blood cell count (RCC) 6400. No organisms are seen on Gram staining. CSF glucose is 3.1 mmol/L (blood glucose 6.4 mmol/L) and protein 0.6 g/L.

Questions

29.3 Should antibiotics be started to treat neurosurgical meningitis before the results of culture are available?

29.4 If started, what initial antibiotics would be appropriate?

Answers

29.3 Should antibiotics be started to treat neurosurgical meningitis before the results of culture are available?

This decision is complicated by the expected elevated CSF cell count consequent to his recent neurosurgical procedure and a borderline low CSF/serum glucose ratio. If this ratio is less than 0.5 then meningitis is more likely but not proven. If there is additional evidence to support intracranial infection such as altered neurological state, wound discharge, or brain imaging showing ventriculitis, antibiotics for neurosurgical meningitis should be commenced. Even without this evidence, there is an argument to treat if he is unstable. If his condition does not mandate immediate treatment, a repeat CSF examination after 24–48 hours would be useful to determine the trend in WCC.

29.4 If started, what initial antibiotics would be appropriate?

Empirical antimicrobials for neurosurgical meningitis/device-related infection should have good central nervous system penetration and target the range of organisms most frequently implicated. For all CSF device-related infections (including those affecting more permanent drainage devices such as ventriculo-peritoneal shunts (VPS)), staphylococci are the most common pathogens (> 50%), with coagulase-negative species (CoNS) accounting for around two-thirds of these isolates. Other skin flora such as propionibacteria account for approximately 10%, Gram-negative rods (including pseudomonas) 8%, and streptococci/enterococci 5% of shunt infections. Fifteen per cent of cultures are polymicrobial and around 10% culture-negative. Isolation of fungi or mycobacteria is rare.

A suitable empirical antibiotic choice might include an intravenous glycopeptide, such as vancomycin, (as an infusion or with loading and maintenance dosing according to weight and renal function, aiming for trough levels of 15–20 mg/l). Parenteral glycopeptides penetrate poorly into the CSF so intrathecal vancomycin via the EVD should be considered if there is a high suspicion of neurosurgical meningitis. Intrathecal antibiotics should be prepared and administered by experienced healthcare professionals to maintain strict asepsis and safe administration.

A broad-spectrum Gram-negative agent that penetrates the central nervous system (CNS), such as cefotaxime or ceftriaxone should also be used. Some local guidelines use Gram-negative agents with additional pseudomonal cover (e.g. ceftazidime).

Case history continued

After 48 hours, *Staphylococcus epidermidis* is grown from the CSF.

Questions

29.5   What changes should be made after the positive culture result?

29.6   Should the EVD be removed?

Answers

29.5 What changes should be made after the positive culture result?

A repeat CSF should be taken, to confirm true *S. epidermidis* shunt infection if possible (less likely if antibiotics were started). The anti-Gram-negative agent can be stopped but the glycopeptide (vancomycin) continued. In cases of methicillin-resistant staphylococcal infections (coagulase negative staphylococci or *Staphylococcus aureus*) intrathecal, in addition to parenteral, vancomycin should be used whilst an EVD is *in situ*.

29.6 Should the EVD be removed?

In proven CSF drain/shunt infection, success rates for treatment with antibiotics alone are poor (< 50%). The EVD should be removed, and, if EVD-dependent, replaced. If possible this should be at a different site. Aseptic repeat CSF sampling for cell count and biochemical parameters should be used to gauge treatment response. The frequency of sampling should be minimized to reduce the chance of new infection. In the scenario described here, common practice is to give a minimum of 7 days antimicrobial treatment after the first negative CSF culture.

Further studies are needed to determine whether, in some cases with low virulence organisms, the drain can be retained and salvage attempted.

Case history continued

His fevers settles and there is a serial improvement in CSF white blood cell count. He completes the planned course of antibiotics and a new EVD is *in situ*, for intracranial pressure management. He is extubated and discharged to the neurosurgical ward. Histology from the pineal mass biopsy lesion reveals germinoma and he commences chemotherapy. Five days after starting this treatment he becomes febrile again and his Glasgow Coma Score drops to 8. He is readmitted to NICU and intubated. Recurrent EVD infection is suspected. CSF examination reveals: WCC 178 (P154 L24), RCC 0 with yeasts seen on Gram stain. *Candida parapsilosis*, subsequently found to be fully susceptible to first-line antifungal agents, is isolated.

Questions

29.7 What anti-infectives should be given now?

29.8 What advice would you give about the subsequent insertion of a shunt?

29.9 How may EVD infections be prevented?

Answers

29.7 What anti-infectives should be given now?

The Infectious Diseases Society of America (IDSA) guidelines recommend intravenous liposomal amphotericin B with or without oral flucytosine in this setting. It is also possible to given amphotericin B intrathecally but there is no evidence to support this practice and it can cause toxicity. As is the case for infection with *Staphylococcus aureus* and Gram-negative bacteria, successful treatment of Candida in this scenario mandates device removal (with re-implantation in a separate site or with a temporary lumbar drain if possible). Antifungal treatment should continue. Common practice is to give at least several weeks of this intravenous antifungal treatment following the first negative CSF culture with serial CSF sampling. Patients should be monitored closely for amphotericin B toxicity (commonly chills, headache, dyspnoea, fever, anaemia, renal impairment, hypokalaemia, hypomagnesemia, and liver function abnormalities). Flucytosine's effects on bone marrow and liver must be carefully monitored, with serum flucytosine levels. Once there is convincing evidence of clinical and CSF response, treatment may be stepped down to oral fluconazole daily as the isolate is susceptible.

29.8 What advice would you give about the subsequent insertion of a shunt?

If the patient requires a permanent neurosurgical shunt this should only be inserted once a negative CSF fungal culture is obtained after completion of treatment. The principles of this two-stage approach (removal of device, use of a temporary device if required, antibiotics, serial CSFs to assess response, stop antibiotics, resample, re-implant new device if no evidence of ongoing infection) can also be applied to infections of other neurosurgical devices such as permanent shunts.

29.9 How may EVD infections be prevented?

Measures to prevent EVD infections include meticulous patient preparation before implantation, good surgical technique, insertion by an experienced practitioner, and good post-operative care. The use of antimicrobial or silver-impregnated EVDs is controversial with mixed studies on their effectiveness.

Further reading

Conen A, Walti LN, Merlo A, Fluckiger U, Battegay M, et al. Characteristics and treatment outcome of cerebrospinal fluid shunt-associated infections in adults: a retrospective analysis of an 11-year period. *Clin Infect Dis* 2008; **47**: 73–82.

Cui Z, Wang B, Zhong Z, Sun Y, Sun Q, et al. Impact of antibiotic- and silver-impregnated external ventricular drains on the risk of infections: a systematic review and meta-analysis. *Am J Infect Control* 2015; **43**: e23–32.

Hepburn-Smith M, Dynkevich I, Spektor M, Lord A, Czeisler B, et al. Establishment of an external ventricular drain best practice guideline: the quest for a comprehensive, universal standard for external ventricular drain care. *J Neurosci Nurs* 2016; **48**: 54–65.

Pappas PG, Kauffman CA, Andes DR, Clancy CJ, Marr KA, et al. Clinical practice guideline for the management of candidiasis: 2016 update by the Infectious Diseases Society of America. *Clin Infect Dis* 2016; **64**: e1–50.

Walti LN, Conen A, Coward J, Jost GF, Trampuz A. Characteristics of infections associated with external ventricular drains of cerebrospinal fluid. *J Infect* 2013; **66**: 424–31.

Case 30

Andrew Woodhouse

Case history

A 35-year-old man with human immunodeficiency virus (HIV) infection is admitted following a generalized seizure. He was diagnosed with HIV infection 8 years ago but struggled to engage with medical services and has not been seen in clinic or taken antiretroviral therapy for 6 years. His family say that over the previous 2 months he has become more withdrawn, seems to have poor concentration, and is less steady on his feet. He has a CD4 lymphocyte count of 45 cells/mm³ and a HIV viral load of over 100,000 copies per ml plasma. An MRI scan has been performed which reports a number of lesions in subcortical white matter which are intense on T2-weighting and do not enhance after gadolinium (Fig. 30.1). The radiologist suggests that the lesions are suggestive of progressive multifocal leucoencephalopathy (PML).

Questions

30.1 What other diagnoses might need to be considered?

30.2 How might a diagnosis of PML be confirmed?

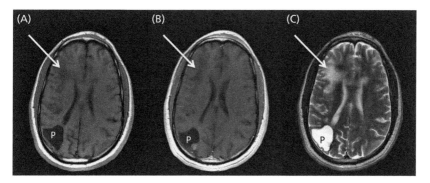

Figure 30.1 MRI scan on presentation. The arrow shows a hypointense lesion on a T1 weighted scan (A) with no enhancement post contrast (B). On T2 weighted image (C) the area is hyperintense. There is no midline shift. The right posterior cystic lesion (P) is long-standing and inactive.

Reproduced courtesy of University Hospitals Birmingham NHS Foundation Trust, UK.

Answers

30.1 What other diagnoses might need to be considered?

In a patient with HIV infection and severe immunosuppression such as the case described, the differential diagnosis of a space occupying cerebral lesion includes toxoplasmosis, cerebral lymphoma, and PML. Imaging appearances alone can suggest a diagnosis of one over the other in some cases but additional tests are often required. In the case of cerebral toxoplasmosis, a suggestive scan followed by a relatively prompt response to anti-toxoplasma therapy is sufficient to make the diagnosis but biopsy is sometimes required.

30.2 How might a diagnosis of PML be confirmed?

PML is an opportunistic infection of the central nervous system caused by the JC polyomavirus (JCV) and is almost always seen in the context of significant immunosuppression. HIV infection is a well-recognized risk factor for developing PML depending on the degree of immunodeficiency. Most patients with HIV and PML have CD4 lymphocyte counts of less than 100 cells/mm^3. MRI findings include multifocal areas of white matter abnormality with hyperintensity on T2-weighted images but low intensity on T1-weighted scans with minimal contrast enhancement. Associated oedema is uncommon. On this basis the diagnosis is suggested by the imaging in the case described. The gold standard of diagnosis would be brain biopsy but this is seldom undertaken. A lumbar puncture should be performed with cerebrospinal fluid (CSF) sent for JCV genome detection by PCR. If positive, this confirms the diagnosis in the appropriate clinical setting with supportive imaging.

Case history continued

CSF examination shows a lymphocyte count of 30/mm^3 and the JCV PCR is positive. The patient is started on antiretroviral therapy (ART) with a combination of tenofovir/emtricitabine/efavirenz. He has a rapid suppression of viral load and an increase in CD4 lymphocyte count to 180 cells/mm^3 over the next 6 weeks. He then develops a deterioration in his balance and his speech becomes slurred. A follow-up MRI scan is arranged which shows areas of oedema around the previously noted areas of demyelination (Fig. 30.2).

Questions

30.3 What treatment for PML can be offered?

30.4 What may explain his subsequent clinical course?

30.5 What treatment may help at this point?

30.6 In addition to HIV infection, in what other circumstances may PML be seen?

30.7 Can PML complicating natalizumab treatment be treated?

30.8 Can PML be prevented?

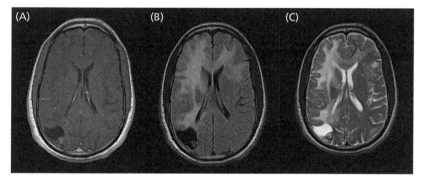

Figure 30.2 MRI scan after 6 weeks antiretroviral treatment. The hypointense lesions on T1 weighted (A) and hyperintense on T2 weighted imaging (C) are more extensive. There is now enhancement on T1 weighted imaging post contrast (B).

Reproduced courtesy of University Hospitals Birmingham NHS Foundation Trust, UK.

Answers

30.3 What treatment for PML can be offered?

There is no proven direct-acting antiviral treatment for JC virus infection. A number of candidate treatments have been suggested but in the small number of trials conducted there has been no convincing evidence of benefit. In patients with HIV infection the most useful intervention is antiretroviral therapy in order to achieve immune recovery and an effective response to JCV. Prior to effective antiretroviral therapy (ART), the 1-year survival after diagnosis of PML was under 10%. In patients able to access effective ART, survival following PML has improved to 50–70% at 1 year.

30.4 What may explain his subsequent clinical course?

He may be experiencing a JCV-related immune reconstitution syndrome (IRIS). IRIS is seen in a number of settings when immune function is restored to an immunocompromised patient. Inflammation results from specific immune responses to the pathogen in question. It is a relatively commonly observed phenomenon in HIV infection and can occur in the context of PML as CD4 +ve T cell recovery occurs with JCV-specific T lymphocytes appearing. MRI changes in PML-related IRIS include the development of contrast enhancement on T1 sequences. Oedema may also be seen. This inflammatory process can lead to clinical features such as headache, focal neurological deficits, and potentially focal or generalized seizures.

30.5 What treatment may help at this point?

Corticosteroids are commonly recommended and used in the treatment of IRIS, complicating HIV treatment due to most underlying causes and this applies to JCV IRIS as well. There is an absence of high-quality evidence to support this approach but it is an accepted treatment. ART is continued and the aim is to control the inflammatory state while continuing to reconstitute the immune system and gain effective immune control of JCV with regression of PML.

30.6 In addition to HIV infection, in what other circumstances may PML be seen?

HIV infection is easily the commonest underlying condition resulting in development of PML. Patients with haematological malignancy can also develop PML and represent the second largest group affected accounting for around 10% of cases in the United States. This group has a particularly poor prognosis due in part to their underlying disease and its treatment but also their inability to reconstitute an effective immune response to JCV. IRIS is seldom seen in such patients and few survive more than a few months after diagnosis.

A more recently recognized group of patients at risk of PML are patients with relapsing-remitting multiple sclerosis (MS) who have been treated with the monoclonal antibody natalizumab. This monoclonal antibody targets α-4 β-1 integrin with resultant inhibition of lymphocyte migration across the blood–brain barrier and this is thought to account for its beneficial effect in MS. JCV-specific lymphocytes are also prevented from entering brain tissue and this loss of immune surveillance is thought to be why PML has been observed in this particular group of patients. PML has been described in a range of other patients receiving immunosuppressive therapy including solid organ transplant recipients and rheumatological patients undergoing immunosuppression but it is relatively uncommon in these settings.

30.7 Can PML complicating natalizumab treatment be treated?

In common with PML complicating HIV infection, the therapeutic approach to PML in the context of natalizumab treatment is to try to restore effective immune function. Stopping the monoclonal accompanied by plasma exchange and immunoadsorption to remove natalizumab allows restoration of lymphocyte migration capacity. This rapid restoration of lymphocyte function and entry into the central nervous system (CNS) may lead to significant JCV IRIS requiring steroid therapy. In addition, the underlying MS may be adversely affected due to removal of lymphocyte blockade and this also needs to be borne in mind.

30.8 Can PML be prevented?

JC virus infection is common and the majority of humans will become infected at some point in their lives. There is no vaccine available and primary infection is asymptomatic. Serology testing for antibody will identify patients previously infected with JC virus and some neurologists looking after patients with MS advocate screening to identify patients at risk of developing PML if given natalizumab.

Seronegative patients can be periodically monitored for development of antibodies as infection in adulthood can occur which will alter their risk profile in terms of developing PML. Seropositive patients may still be offered natalizumab treatment although some centres would recommend frequent MRI scans with the aim of detecting early subclinical lesions of PML which can then allow discontinuation of antibody therapy.

In HIV infection the aim is early diagnosis of HIV infection prior to significant immune system deterioration. Effective ART can then be started prior to significant declines in CD4 count making development of PML and of PML IRIS unlikely outcomes.

Further reading

Cinque P, Koralnik IJ, Gerevini S, Miro JM, Price RW. Progressive multifocal leukoencephalopathy complicating HIV-1 infection. *Lancet Infect Dis* 2009; **9**: 625–36.

Clifford DB. Progressive multifocal leukoencephalopathy therapy. *J Neurovirol* 2015; **21**: 632–6.

Curruthers R, Berger J. Progressive multifocal leukoencephalopthy and JC Virus-related disease in modern neurology practice. *Mult Scler Relat Disord* 2014: **3**; 419–30.

Pavlovic D, Patera A, Nyberg F, Gerber M, Liu M, et al. Progressive multifocal leukoencephalopathy: current treatment options and future perspectives. *Ther Adv Neurol Disord*. 2015: **8**; 255–73.

Tan CS, Koralnik IJ. Beyond progressive multifocal leukoencephalopathy: expanded pathogenesis of JC virus infection in the central nervous system. *Lancet Neurol* 2010; **9**: 425–37.

Section 6

Systemic infections

Case 31

Andrew Woodhouse

Case history

A 37-year-old woman is referred for evaluation of fever and a neutrophil leukocytosis with no response to broad-spectrum antibiotics. Four weeks previously she developed a sore throat, fever, and pain in a number of joints. A non-itching pink rash was noted over her arms and upper torso, particularly when she had fever. Initially she was felt to have a viral infection and she was managed symptomatically. Over the first 3 weeks of her illness she attended her General Practitioner (GP) twice and the Emergency Department (ED) once because of persisting fever and feeling unwell. Her temperature was intermittently as high as 39.1 °C. Over the previous week she has been an inpatient. Her chest X-ray (CXR) revealed a possible infiltrate and she was started on co-amoxiclav, subsequently changed to pipericillin/tazobactam due to persisting fever. Blood and urine cultures are negative, C-reactive protein (CRP) is high at 268 mg/L, and her liver enzymes are mildly raised in a hepatocellular pattern. Her neutrophil count is 10.8 and she has a normochromic anemia but the remainder of the full blood count (FBC) is normal. A computerized tomography (CT) scan of thorax and abdomen has not found any significant abnormality and in particular, no evidence of pneumonia.

A number of other investigations are obtained. Further blood cultures are negative. The rash and arthralgia has raised the question of a connective tissue disorder. Autoantibodies are negative but her ferritin is markedly elevated at > 40,000 µg/l. A bone marrow examination reports a minor degree of haemophagocytosis.

Questions

31.1 Does this patient have a PUO?

31.2 How should you initially approach the problem of PUO?

31.3 What diagnosis needs to be considered here?

31.4 What treatment should be given?

31.5 What proportion of cases of PUO are due to infection?

31.6 What are the most useful investigations for PUO?

31.7 What is the prognosis for undiagnosed PUO?

Answers

31.1 Does this patient have a PUO?

Yes. The classical definition of PUO was laid out by Petersdorf and Beeson in the early 1960s. They defined it as a fever above 38.3 °C on at least 3 occasions with a duration of illness of 3 weeks including a week of hospital-based investigation without a diagnosis being reached. In the subsequent decades it has been recognized that the original definition can be modified according to patient group and the healthcare setting where the patient is being evaluated. PUO has been separately characterized, for example, in patients with HIV infection, organ transplant recipients, returning travellers, and nosocomial onset. Also, with the shift toward out-patient medicine, a strict period of in-hospital investigation is not necessarily required to meet the criteria. The cardinal features remain a documented fever (> 38.3 °C) on more than 2 occasions over a period of 3 weeks and no diagnosis despite a reasonable range of investigations. The patient described clearly meets the classical description and can justifiably be described as a PUO. There is a tendency in modern practice to label any patient with a fever in whom the cause in not known after a brief initial evaluation and investigations as a PUO but this should be avoided.

31.2 How should you initially approach the problem of PUO?

A PUO evaluation requires an open mind and a systematic approach. Throughout the evaluation, the emphasis should be on seeking clues to direct investigation as much as possible rather than adopting an unfocused approach.

History

This can play an enormous role in directing efforts, not just in terms of any localizing symptoms and their pattern and duration but also seeking any potential exposures through travel, recreation, or occupation that might suggest certain infections. Drug and family history are also important and whether any interventions have made a difference to symptoms.

Examination

This should be undertaken with careful attention to examining the eyes, oral cavity, assessing for peripheral lymphadenopathy, examining joints, and reviewing the skin for signs of rash. In the case described, empiric broad-spectrum antibiotics have been given with little positive effect and stopping them is appropriate in the context of ongoing observation and investigation.

31.3 What diagnosis needs to be considered here?

Clinically she meets criteria for a diagnosis of adult-onset Stills disease (AOSD) due to fever, leukocytosis, rash, duration of symptoms, and arthralgia. The mild hepatitis is also consistent and although not part of the diagnostic criteria, marked hyperferritinaemia is highly suggestive. High ferritin levels are seen in other inflammatory states including haemophagocytic lymphohistiocytosis (HLH), a macrophage-activation disorder which was also a consideration in the case described here. However, the degree of haemophagocytosis in bone marrow was relatively mild. Haemophagocytosis is sometimes seen in AOSD.

31.4 What treatment should be given?

Treatment for AOSD is based on anti-inflammatory strategies. In mild cases, non-steroidal anti-inflammatory drugs may be sufficient but frequently steroids are required to suppress inflammation and improve symptoms. In this case, 40 mg of prednisolone was commenced with resolution of fever within 2–3 days. Steroids were gradually tapered and over a 3-month period, she made a full recovery and her inflammatory markers returned to normal.

31.5 What proportion of cases of PUO are due to infection?

Infectious aetiologies account for a minority of the causes of PUO in most large recent series. Typically, less than a third of cases are proven to be due to infection. The other major diagnostic groups are malignancy and non-infectious inflammatory disorders, including auto-immune, auto-inflammatory, and vasculitic disorders. The proportion due to infection tend to be higher in series published from resource-limited countries. In resource-rich settings the widespread availability of antibiotics has reduced the incidence of chronic bacterial infections and many infectious diseases such as tuberculosis have become relatively less common. Despite the tendency to equate new onset of fever with an infectious cause it is important to be aware of the wide array of non-infection conditions which can cause fever and to investigate appropriately if initial symptoms and signs suggest these.

31.6 What are the most useful investigations for PUO?

In a febrile patient with or without abnormal findings on examination or clues in the history, the investigation pathway requires careful consideration.

- Initial investigations should include routine haematology and biochemistry including inflammatory markers, liver function tests, and autoantibodies.
- Cultures should be taken including blood and urine and other samples as indicated by apparent organ involvement.
- Serology tests should be selectively requested depending on history including travel and residence in other parts of the world.

◆ Imaging can be extremely useful with computerized tomography (CT) scan of thorax and abdomen and pelvis often undertaken to look for cryptic foci of bacterial infection, potential tuberculosis, or evidence of malignancy. Recently there has been interest in the use of ^{18}F-FDG-PET-CT (^{10}F-fluorodeoxyglucose-Positron Emission Tomography-Computerized Tomography) in cases of PUO, including its use early in the course of investigation. Fig. 31.1 is a PET-CT image showing high uptake in upper abdominal lymph nodes which were not obvious

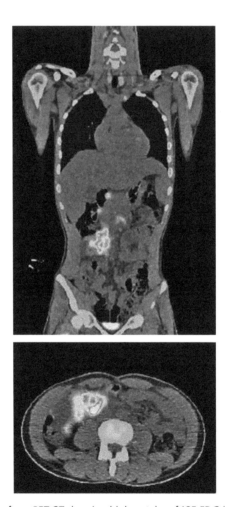

Figure 31.1 Images from PET-CT showing high uptake of ^{1}8F-FDG in upper abdominal lymph nodes in a patient with fever of 8 weeks duration. No other lymphadenopathy was evident. Tuberculosis was diagnosed by histology and culture after biopsy samples obtained (see colour plate).

on initial plain CT. Tuberculosis was subsequently diagnosed on biopsy samples. It can be particularly helpful in terms of detecting malignant disease and vasculitis in addition to possible infective foci but its role in work-up of PUO is still evolving. In most settings it is considered part of a second-line round of investigations when diagnosis remains elusive.

◆ Bone marrow biopsy is potentially helpful, particularly when there is concern about an underlying haematological cause for fever. In the diagnosis of infection it can be useful for a small subset of patients with appropriate exposure history looking to visualize, detect by molecular methods, or culture organisms that can be otherwise elusive such as brucella and leishmania. It is not an investigation that should be applied routinely.

31.7 What is the prognosis for undiagnosed PUO?

Despite intensive and repeated investigation, up to a third of patients with PUO remain without a formal diagnosis. In general, the prognosis for patients with undiagnosed PUO after thorough investigation is good with low mortality. Symptoms extending beyond a year are seldom eventually attributed to infection or malignancy. A high proportion of patients whose PUO eludes diagnosis spontaneously remit with time but a prolonged period of monitoring may be required and any change in symptoms or signs merits a review of all investigations to date and further targeted evaluation.

Further reading

Brown M. Pyrexia of unknown origin 90 years on: a paradigm of modern clinical medicine. *Postgrad Med J* 2015; **91**: 665–9.

Crouzet, J, Boudousq V, Lechliche C, Poujet JP, Kotzi PO, et al. Place of ^{18}F-FDG-PET with computed tomography in the diagnostic algorithm of patients with fever of unknown origin. *Eur J Clin Microbiol Infect Dis* 2012; **31**: 1727–33.

Cunha BA, Lortholary O, Cunha CB. Fever of unknown origin: a clinical approach. *Am J Med* 2015; **128**: 1138e1–e15.

Dibble EH, Yoo DC, Noto RB. Role of PET/CT in workup of fever without a source. *Radiographics* 2016; **36**: 1166–76.

Mulders-Manders C, Simon A, Bleeker-Rovers C. Fever of unknown origin. *Clinical Med* 2015; **15**: 280–4.

Case 32

Maheshi Ramasamy

Case history

A 42-year-old woman with a tunnelled dual lumen vascular haemodialysis catheter develops a fever whilst on dialysis. There is no evidence of tunnel or exit site infection. Blood cultures taken from the haemodialysis circuit and from a peripheral blood sample grow *Staphylococcus epidermidis* in all four blood culture bottles, susceptible to vancomycin.

Questions

32.1 Should the infected catheter be removed immediately?

32.2 How should this haemodialysis catheter infection be managed?

Answers

32.1 Should the infected catheter be removed immediately?

No. For catheter infections caused by coagulase-negative staphylococci and for some Gram-negative bacteria, which are less likely to develop biofilms, catheter salvage may be attempted. For catheter infections caused by biofilm-forming organisms such as *Pseudomonas* spp. it is recommended that the vascular catheter is removed, and a temporary non-tunnelled catheter inserted at a distant site. If no alternative sites are present for catheter insertion, then the infected catheter may be exchanged over a guidewire. However, regardless of the infecting organism, patients with haemodialysis catheter-related infections with haemodynamic instability, persistent bloodstream infection (BSI) after initiation of appropriate antibiotics, or evidence of tunnel tract infection should have their catheter removed.

32.2 How should this haemodialysis catheter infection be managed?

The patient should be treated with antibiotics that can be administered with haemodialysis, such as vancomycin, to avoid the necessity of further vascular catheter insertion in dialysis patients whose peripheral veins may be required for the formation of fistulae and grafts. For a low virulence, low biofilm-producing organism such as *Staphylococcus epidermidis*, antibiotic therapy may be given for 2 weeks.

Infection in vascular catheters which have been *in situ* for longer than 2 weeks, and without evidence of exit site or tunnel infection, is largely due to intra-luminal infection, with bacteria growing in biofilms along the lumen rather than in free-living planktonic states. Antibiotic locks involve filling the lumen of catheters with supra-therapeutic concentrations of drugs to eradicate this bacterial biofilm during attempted line salvage. Locks may contain a variety of antimicrobial agents such as vancomycin, gentamicin, ceftazidime, or ethanol, mixed with heparin or normal saline. The use of antibiotic locks is associated with higher rates of line salvage, although their success is dependent on the infecting organism. Antibiotic concentrations decrease in the catheter lumen over time, therefore antibiotic locks should be changed every 48 hours (e.g. on haemodialysis) and should be used for 2 weeks.

Case history continued

Subsequently, a month later she develops rigors and has erythema and tenderness around the catheter insertion site. Blood cultures are taken and from both bottles, a methicillin-susceptible *Staphylococcus aureus* is isolated at 18 hours. She defervesces after 36 hours of antibiotics.

Question

32.3   What should the further management of this patient be?

Answer

32.3 What should the further management of this patient be?

S. aureus is a common cause of nosocomial BSI. Repeat blood cultures should be taken at 48 hours after commencing anti-staphylococcal antibiotics to ensure the patient does not have persistent BSI, which is highly predictive of complicated or metastatic infection. The patient should be re-examined regularly for secondary foci, for example, bone/joint pain. The incidence of endocarditis in *S. aureus* blood-stream infection (SABSI) is reported at between 10–30% and all patients with SABSI should be assessed clinically for evidence of endocarditis. Patients who are *low risk* for endocarditis are those who have line-related SABSI with no permanent intra cardiac device and are not on haemodialysis. They defervesce rapidly with no evidence of a secondary focus or stigmata of endocarditis. In these patients it is reasonable practice to treat with no echocardiogram. All patients with SABSI who *do not* fall into this low-risk group should have urgent echocardiography (ideally a trans-oesophageal echocardiogram). In all cases of SABSI blood cultures should be repeated at 48–72 hours and, if positive, an urgent echocardiogram and search for any other focus is warranted.

In the absence of a secondary focus, intravenous anti-staphylococcal antibiotics (e.g. flucloxacillin or an anti-staphylococcal cephalosporin) should be administered. There are no clinical trials on the duration of antimicrobials, but common practice is to treat for 14 days.

Case history continued

One year later, she is admitted to intensive care having sustained severe abdominal trauma requiring a hemicolectomy and stoma formation. She is treated for a ventilator acquired pneumonia with a 5-day course of piperacillin-tazobactam. Ten days into her hospital admission, she develops a fever and becomes hypotensive. She has a central venous line in her right internal jugular vein for administration of fluids and total parenteral nutrition, the entry site of which appears clean and uninflamed. Paired peripheral and central line blood cultures are sent and these both flag positive at 12 hours. Gram staining reveals a yeast like organism in 2 out of 2 peripheral and 2 out of 2 central catheter blood culture bottles, and Gram-positive cocci in 1 out of 2 of the central catheter samples. These are subsequently identified as a *Candida albicans* and a *S. epidermidis*, respectively.

Questions

32.4 What is the significance of these isolates?

32.5 What is the management of catheter associated candidaemia in this patient?

32.4 What is the significance of these isolates?

Candida spp. in blood cultures in unlikely to be a contaminant and is highly suggestive of catheter-associated candidaemia (Boxes 32.1 and 32.2). However, *S. epidermidis* may represent a contaminant skin-commensal organism or line colonization, as it is present in only half of all central catheter samples and not in peripheral samples. Unless there is evidence of persistent *S. epidermidis* BSI or the patient has prosthetic intravascular or orthopaedic devices, it should be disregarded. Distinguishing between pathogenic and contaminant isolates may require quantitative sampling (Box 32.1). This relies on equivalent volume sampling of peripheral and catheter hub blood, which is difficult to achieve in clinical practice.

32.5 What is the management of catheter-associated candidaemia in this patient?

As *Candida* spp. tend to form biofilms on prosthetic materials, this patient's central venous catheter should be removed. *C. albicans* is the commonest species and is normally susceptible to azoles (unless already exposed to these agents), echinocandins, and amphotericin B. Fluconazole is favoured for tolerability and high bioavailability and is given as an 800 mg loading dose, followed by 400 mg daily (modified if there is renal dysfunction). There is a rising prevalence of non-albicans isolates including *C. glabrata* and *C. krusei* with decreased susceptibility to azoles—invasive infections

---

Box 32.1 Microbiological criteria for diagnosis of intravascular catheter associated infection

♦ Same organism grown from *at least* 1 peripheral blood culture *and* from a culture of the catheter tip*

OR

♦ Same organism grown from *both* a catheter hub blood sample *and* a peripheral vein blood sample using quantitative[†] or differential time to positivity (DTP)[§] criteria.

*Growth of >15 colony-forming units (cfu) from a 5-cm segment of the catheter tip by semi-quantitative (roll-plate) culture or growth of > 10^2 cfu from a catheter by a quantitative (sonication) broth culture. Catheter tips should not be routinely cultured on line removal, but only when infection is suspected, in conjunction with blood cultures.

[†] A colony count of microbes grown from blood obtained through the catheter hub that is at least threefold greater than the colony count from blood obtained from a peripheral vein.

[§] Growth of microbes from a blood sample drawn from a catheter hub at least 2 hours before microbial growth is detected in a blood sample obtained from a peripheral vein.

Adapted with permission from Mermel, LA, et al. (2009). Clinical practice guidelines for the diagnosis and management of intravascular catheter-related infection: 2009 Update by the Infectious Diseases Society of America. *Clin Infect Dis* 49(1): 1–45. DOI: 10.1086/599376.

> **Box 32.2 Risk factors for Candidaemia**
>
> ◆ Adult intensive care unit (ICU) admission
> ◆ Total parenteral nutrition
> ◆ Broad-spectrum antibiotics
> ◆ Recipient of solid organ/bone marrow transplant
> ◆ Chemotherapy, particularly regimens associated with mucositis
> ◆ Burns
> ◆ Central venous catheters
> ◆ Prior surgery, particularly abdominal surgery
>
> Source: data from Kullberg BJ and Arendrup MC (2015). Invasive Candidiasis. *N Engl J Med* 373(15):1445–56. DOI: 10.1056/NEJMra1315399.

with these species can usually be treated with an echinocandin when there is no central nervous system or urinary focus. Follow-up blood cultures should be performed daily or every other day to establish clearance. Common practice is to treat until 2 weeks after resolution of candidaemia.

All patients with candidaemia should be assessed for metastatic infection. Observational studies suggest up to 8% of patients with candidaemia have endocarditis and echocardiography should be performed routinely. Furthermore, ocular candidiasis can occur in 16% of patients, presenting either as chorioretinitis or endophthalmitis. All patients should therefore have dilated fundoscopy, preferably by an ophthalmologist, within the first week of treatment.

Further reading

Arechabala MC, Catoni MI, Claro JC, Rojas NP, Rubio ME, et al. Antimicrobial lock solutions for preventing catheter-related infections in haemodialysis. *Cochrane Database of Systemic Reviews* 2018; 4: CD010597.

Joseph JP, Meddows TR, Webster DP, Newton JD, Myerson SG, et al. Prioritizing echocardiography in *Staphylococcus aureus* bacteraemia. *J Antimicr Chemother* 2013; **68**: 444–9.

Holland TL, Arnold C, Fowler VG Jr. Clinical management of *Staphylococcus aureus* bacteremia: a review. *JAMA* 2014; **312**: 1330–41.

Mermel LA, Allon M, Bouza E, Craven DE, Flynn P, et al. Clinical practice guidelines for the diagnosis and management of intravascular catheter-related infection: 2009 Update by the Infectious Diseases Society of America. *Clin Infect Dis.* 2009; **49**: 1–45. doi: 10.1086/599376.

Pappas PG, Kauffman CA, Andes DR, Clancy CJ, Marr KA, et al. Clinical practice guideline for the management of candidiasis: 2016 update by the Infectious Diseases Society of America. *Clin Infect Dis* 2016; **15**: 409–17. doi: 10.1093/cid/civ1194.

Case 33

T H Nicholas Wong

Case history

A 50-year-old man presents to his local hospital with a 4-week history of chest discomfort and shortness of breath. He also reports a 4-month history of fatigue and intermittent fever. There is no history of smoking, alcohol use, or intravenous drug use. He worked as a farmer tending livestock. Physical examination demonstrates a loud grade III/IV diastolic murmur heard along the right sternal border with radiation to the carotid arteries bilaterally. On respiratory examination, there are a few bilateral inspiratory wheezes. He has a conjunctival haemorrhage and 2 Janeway lesions. Trans-thoracic echocardiogram reveals a vegetation on the inferior cusp of the aortic valve. Three sets of blood cultures are sent before empiric antibiotic administration but are sterile at 7 days.

Questions

33.1 What is the diagnosis and how is it defined?

33.2 What are the risk factors?

33.3 What additional questions should be sought when taking a history?

33.4 Can endocarditis be non-infective in origin?

33.5 What microbiological pathogens can cause this condition?

33.6 How can the diagnosis be optimized?

33.7 What are the treatment options?

Answers

33.1 What is the diagnosis and how is it defined?

Based on the echocardiographic findings, fever, and vasculitic phenomena, this patient has infective endocarditis (IE) using modified Dukes Criteria.

Blood culture-negative infective endocarditis (BCNIE) is defined as endocarditis without known aetiology following inoculation of at least 3 independent blood samples in a standard blood culture system and negative cultures after 5 days of incubation and sub-culturing.

Cultures are negative in infectious endocarditis for three major reasons:

1. Previous administration of antimicrobial agents

2. Inadequate microbiological techniques

3. Infection with highly fastidious bacteria or non-bacterial pathogens

BCNIE can occur in up to 31% of all cases of infective endocarditis and most commonly arises as a consequence of recent antibiotics

33.2 What are the risk factors?

Risk factors for BCNIE include recent antimicrobial use, exposure to fastidious organisms including zoonotic agents, underlying valvular heart disease, and the presence of a pacemaker. No convincing evidence exists to show that endocarditis involving any particular valve (e.g. tricuspid) is more likely to be culture negative.

33.3 What additional questions should be sought when taking a history?

The history should cover the following questions:

- Recent antimicrobials
- Recent hospital admissions
- Intravascular lines, evidence of any line infections
- Presence of a pacemaker or prosthetic valve
- Immunosuppression, including HIV infection (fungi, *Coxiella* spp.)
- Ingestion of unpasteurized milk, cheese, or insufficiently cooked meat and/or travel to the Middle East, Mediterranean, or other endemic areas (*Brucella* spp.)
- Contact with or occupational exposure to farm animals, particularly to their products of conception or significant exposure to an abattoir—as in this patient (*Coxiella* spp.)
- Contact with the human body louse, homeless shelters or chronic alcoholism (*Bartonella quintana*)

◆ Cat contact or ownership (*Bartonella henselae*)

◆ Laboratory exposure to pathogens (e.g. *Histoplasma* spp., *Coxiella* spp.).

33.4 Can endocarditis be non-infective in origin?

Yes. Non-bacterial thrombotic endocarditis (NBTE) is a form of endocarditis where small sterile vegetations are deposited on the valve leaflets, formerly known as marantic endocarditis. A history of inflammatory/connective tissue disease such as rheumatic fever or systemic lupus erythematosis (SLE) should also be sought. NBTE associated with SLE is known as Libman–Sacks endocarditis. A history of hypercoagulable states, malignant cancers, especially mucin-producing adenocarcinomas, and catheter trauma should be sought as these can mimic endocarditis.

33.5 What microbiological pathogens can cause this condition?

When the patient has received recent antimicrobials, the range of organisms causing BCNIE is similar to that in culture-positive endocarditis, that is, viridans streptococci, enterococci, and, less commonly, staphylococci or HACEK organisms (see following). When there is *no* history of recent antimicrobials other groups of organisms should be considered as follows;

◆ *HACEK group of organisms*: Organisms belonging to the HACEK group (Table 33.1) are part of the normal oropharyngeal flora. They require enriched media (e.g. chocolate agar), grow in atmospheres with 5% CO_2, and account for a small number (5–10%) of cases of endocarditis. In BCNIE, blood culture incubation should always be prolonged for at least 14 days

◆ *Other fastidious organisms*: These may include:

• Nutritionally variant streptococci requiring media supplemented with either pyridoxal or cysteine for growth

Table 33.1 Organisms in the HACEK group

H	Traditionally this is *Haemophilus aphrophilus* (subsequently called *Aggregatibacter aphrophilus* and *Aggregatibacter paraphrophilus*) but many *Haemophilus* spp. can cause human infections
A	*Actinobacillus actinomycetemcomitans* (subsequently called *Aggregatibacter actinomycetemcomitans*)
C	*Cardiobacterium hominis* (and other *Cardiobacterium* spp. e.g. *K. valvarum*)
E	*Eikenella corrodens*
K	*Kingella kingae* (and other *Kingella* spp. e.g. *K. denitrificans, K. potus*)

- *Brucella* spp. (which have similar growth characteristics to HACEK organisms). If suspected, all specimens and blood culture isolates should be examined in a containment level 3 facility using a class 1 biosafety cabinet.
- *Bartonella* spp. (low prevalence 1% in northern Europe and the United Kingdom, higher in southern Europe and North Africa)
- *Coxiella burnetti*
- Fungi, e.g.
  - with total parental nutrition (TPN) lines or other long-term vascular access—*Candida* spp.
  - in immunocompromised hosts: *Candida* spp., *Aspergillus* spp., *Mucor* spp.
- *Tropheryma whipplei*
- *Legionella pneumophila*
- *Mycoplasma* spp.
- *Mycobacterium tuberculosis* and non-tuberculous mycobacteria (NTMs)

33.6 How can the microbiological diagnosis be optimized?

Diagnostic tests for culture-negative endocarditis include histopathological evaluation of valvular tissue when surgical excision is performed, molecular techniques (polymerase chain reaction), serologic assays, and special culture techniques (e.g. shell vial and lysis centrifugation). In all cases, appropriate precautions should be taken with specimen and culture handling. *Brucella* and *Coxiella* spp. are in Category 3 of the Advisory Committee on Dangerous Pathogens (ACDP) human pathogen hazard group.

Histopathology

Special tissue staining (Gram, Giemsa, acid-fast, Warthin–Starry, and Periodic acid-Schiff [PAS] stains) of explanted valve tissue can be useful for pathogen identification of infectious endocarditis as well as non-infectious mimickers including NBTE, rheumatic endocarditis, or atrial myxoma.

Polymerase chain reaction (PCR)

Molecular testing of excised valve material may be useful for cases in which there is a high clinical suspicion of IE but a definitive microbiological diagnosis has not been possible to establish with culture or serology. This is particularly valuable in patients with previous antibiotic exposure, since bacterial DNA frequently persists even when organisms are present in quantities too low to be detected via culture.

There are broad-range PCR techniques for amplifying 16SrDNA (for bacteria) or 18SrDNA (for fungi), which can then be sequenced for pathogen identification. The most frequently identified bacteria have included streptococci, staphylococci,

Bartonella spp., and *T. whipplei*. In addition, there are real-time PCR techniques for diagnosis of specific pathogens including *Bartonella* spp., *C. burnetii* (Q fever), and *Tropheryma whipplei*.

Serological assays

The aetiologic agents in culture-negative IE that may be identified by serology include *Coxiella burnetii, Bartonella* spp., *Legionella* spp., and *Brucella* spp. *Coxiella burnetii* phase I antibody titres > 800 are diagnostic for Q fever endocarditis. The presence of IgG (immunoglobulin G) antiphospholipid during acute Q fever is predictive of evolution to endocarditis. Bartonella IgG levels ≥ 800 are diagnostic for *Bartonella* spp. However, patients with Q fever may have low-level cross-reacting antibodies to *Bartonella* spp. and/or *Chlamydia* spp. Furthermore, the role of *Chlamydia* spp. in the aetiology of IE is controversial and difficult to ascertain because of the cross-reacting antibodies to *Bartonella* spp.

Special culture techniques

These have mostly been superseded in routine practice by molecular techniques. Lysis centrifugation can improve yield of fastidious organisms (e.g. *Brucella* spp. and fungi). This culture system contains components that lyse leukocytes and erythrocytes, as well as inactivate plasma complement and certain antibiotics. The cell lysis allows release of intracellular microorganisms, and the centrifugation step concentrates the organisms, which can then be plated directly onto supportive medium.

Shell vial cell culture

Shell vial cell culture assay of blood or excised heart valves allows the isolation of *Coxiella burnetii, Bartonella* spp., *T. whipplei*, and *Brucella* spp. and has been useful in identifying the etiologic agent in culture-negative infective endocarditis. This technique is restricted to specialized laboratories and is being superseded by molecular diagnostics.

33.7 What are the treatment options?

There should be early discussion about the role and the timing of valvular surgery in patients with endocarditis. It is beyond the scope of this setting to discuss surgical criteria.

Antimicrobial therapy should be directed when possible and prolonged in most cases. Patients with culture-negative endocarditis should be divided into 2 groups, assuming appropriate microbiology cultures and specimen processing has occurred.

- *Group 1*. Those who received antimicrobial therapy before collection of blood cultures. For those with acute presentation coverage for *S. aureus* should be included. For more indolent presentations, coverage of viridans streptococci

Table 33.2 Antibiotic treatment of blood culture-negative infective endocarditis

Pathogens	Proposed therapy[a]	Treatment outcome
Brucella spp.	Doxycycline (200 mg/24 h) plus cotrimoxazole (960 mg/12 h) plus rifampin (300–600 mg/24 h) for ≥3–6 months[b] orally	Treatment success defined as an antibody titre <1:60. Some authors recommend adding gentamicin for the first 3 weeks.
C. burnetii (agent of Q fever)	Doxycycline (200 mg/24 h) plus hydroxycholoroquine (200–600 mg/64 h)[c] orally (> 18 months of treatment)	Treatment success defined as anti-phase I IgG titre <1:200, and IgA and IgM titres <1:50.
Bartonella spp.[d]	Doxycycline 100 mg/12 h orally for 4 weeks plus gentamicin (3 mg/24 h) i.v. for 2 weeks	Treatment success expected in ≥90%.
Legionella spp.	Levofloxacin (500 mg/12 h) i.v. or orally for ≥6 weeks or clarithromycin (500 mg/12 h) i.v. for 2 weeks, then orally for 4 weeks plus rifampin (300–1200 mg/24 h)	Optimal treatment unknown.
Mycoplasma spp.	Levofloxacin (500 mg/12 h) i.v. or orally for ≥6 months[e]	Optimal treatment unknown.
T. whipplei (agent of Whipple's disease)[f]	Doxycycline (200 mg/24 h) plus hydroxycholoroquine (200–600 mg/24 h)[c] orally for ≥18 months	Long-term treatment, optimal duration unknown.

ID = infectious disease; IE = infective endocarditis; ig = immunoglobulin; i.v. = intravenous; U = units.

[a]Owing to the lack of large series, the optimal duration of treatment of IE due to these pathogens is unknown. The presented durations are based on selected case reports.

Consulation with an ID specialist is recommended.

[b]Addition of streptomycin (15 mg/kg/24 in 2 doses) for the first few weeks is optional.

[c]Doxycycline plus hydroxychloroquine (with monitoring of serum hydroxycyclocine levels) is significantly superior to doxycycline.[194]

[d]Several therapeutic regimens have been reported, including aminopencillins (ampicillin or amoxicillin, 12g/24 h i.v.) or cephalosporins (ceftriaxone, 2g/24 h i.v) combined with aminoglycosides (gentamicin or netilmicin).[195] Dosages are as for streptococcal and enterococcal IE (*Tables 16* and *18*).[196],[197]

[e]Newer fluoroquinolones (levofloxacin, moxifloxacin) are more potent than ciprofloxacin against intracellular pathogens such as *Mycoplasma* spp. '*Legionella* spp.' and *Chlamydia* spp.

[f]Treatment of Whipple's IE remains highly empirical. In the case of central nervous system involvement, sulfadiazine 1.5 g/6 h orally must be added to doxycycline. An alternative therapy is ceftriaxone (2 g/24 h i.v.) for 2–4 weeks or pencillin G (2 million U/4 h) and streptomycin (1 g/24 h) i.v. for 2–4 weeks followed by cotrimoxazole (800 mg/12 h) orally. Trimethoprim is not active against *T. whipplei*. Successes have been reported with long-term therapy (>1 year).

Adapted from Habib G, et al. (2015). 2015 ESC Guidelines for the management of infective endocarditis: The Task Force for the Management of Infective Endocarditis of the European Society of Cardiology (ESC). Endorsed by: European Association for Cardio-Thoracic Surgery (EACTS), the European Association of Nuclear Medicine (EANM). *Eur Heart J* 21:36(44):3075–3128. DOI: 10.1093/eurheartj/ehv319. Source: data from Brouqui P and Raoult D (2001). Endocarditis due to rare and fastidious bacteria. *Clin Microbiol Rev* 14:177–207. DOI: 10.1128/CMR.14.1.177–207.2001.

and enterococci should be given. Therapy for HACEK organisms should be considered. When a prosthetic valve is present, cover for methicillin-resistant *S. aureus* and coagulase-negative staphylococci should be included.

◆ *Group 2*. Those who have *not* received prior antimicrobial therapy may have infections caused by uncommon or rare endocarditis pathogens that do not grow in routinely used blood culture systems. Empiric treatment is difficult unless the causative pathogen can be identified. The European guidelines for specific unusual infections are included in Table 33.2.

Further reading

2015 ESC Guidelines for the management of infective endocarditis : The Task Force for the management of infective endocarditis of the European Society of Cardiology (ESC). *Eur Heart J* 2015; **36**: 3075–128. doi: 10.1093/eurheartj/ehv319. Epub 2015 Aug 29.

Brouqui P, Raoult D. Endocarditis due to rare and fastidious bacteria. *Clin Microbiol Rev* 2001; **14**: 177.

Li JS, Sexton DJ, Mick N, Nettles R, Fowler Jr VG., et al. Proposed modifications to the Duke Criteria for the diagnosis of infective endocarditis. *Clin Infect Dis* 2000; **30**: 633–8.

Baddour LM, Wilson WR, Bayer AS, Fowler VG, Bolger AF, et al. AHA scientific statement, infective endocarditis. *Circulation* 2005; **111**: e394–e434.

Vondracek M, Sartipy U, Aufwerber E, Julander I, Lindblom D, et al. 16S rDNA sequencing of valve tissue improves microbiological diagnosis in surgically treated patients with infective endocarditis. *J Infect* 2011; **62**: 472.

Case 34

Hilary Humphreys

Case history

A 57-year-old man undergoes emergency surgery for a ruptured abdominal aortic aneurysm and post-operatively he is transferred to the general intensive care unit (ICU). He had a colon resection 2 years previously for cancer. He regularly travels to Asia where he was hospitalized during the preceding year for pneumonia. Four days after surgery, he spikes a temperature of 39.5 °C, develops hypotension requiring inotropic support, and his abdomen becomes distended. The surgical team take blood cultures and start him on intravenous cefotaxime and metronidazole. The following day, the patient is still acutely septic, requiring increased nor-adrenaline, and he remains pyrexial despite the addition of gentamicin. Gram-negative bacilli are seen on microscopy in the blood cultures.

Questions

34.1 How likely are positive blood cultures in this setting?

34.2 How appropriate is the choice of antibiotics?

34.3 Why might the patient not be responding to cefotaxime and metronidazole?

Answers

34.1 How likely are positive blood cultures in this setting?

Around 5–10% of blood cultures taken for any reason are positive but in patients with septic shock, the proportion is about 50%. However, 15–30% of all isolates from positive blood cultures are contaminants. The higher the blood volume collected the higher the yield; the yield is 61% from the first set of blood cultures, 78% from the first two sets, and 93% from three sets of blood cultures. To optimize this in the ICU, 10 ml of blood should be inoculated into each bottle, that is, approximately 20 ml for 1 set of 2 bottles. Ideally when more than 1 blood culture set is taken, there should be a time interval between them. Blood should be taken via central lines as well as from a peripheral vein if intravascular-catheter-related bloodstream infection (BSI) is suspected, and all blood cultures should be incubated within four hours.

34.2 How appropriate is the choice of antibiotics?

The chosen combination covers most abdominal aerobic Gram-negative bacilli (AGNB) and anaerobes. However, many healthcare-acquired AGNB will not be susceptible to third-generation cephalosporins such as cefotaxime, and this may be especially so for this patient who has been an in-patient for four days with a background of hospitalization abroad.

34.3 Why might the patient not be responding to cefotaxime and metronidazole?

Cefotaxime is inactivated by extended-spectrum β-lactamases (ESBL), enzymes that hydrolyse penicillins and cephalosporins (see Case 15). There are three groups of ESLBs: TEM, SHV, and CTX-M. CTX-M β-lactamases are the commonest, of which there are more than 50 types. *E. coli* and *K. pneumomiae* are the major ESBL producers worldwide. As these enzymes are associated with mobile genetic elements, they can spread widely and are often associated with resistance to other antibiotics such as the aminoglycosides. Cefotaxime resistance can also result from changes in the expression of intrinsic chromosomal genes (ampC) in some species, notably *Enterobacter* spp. and *Serratia* spp.

A further reason for ongoing sepsis may be a persistent source for the BSI, such as abdominal abscess, as the patient had abdominal surgery 4 days earlier and for which source control is essential. It is also possible that there is an infection at another site such as the chest or device, that is, intravascular.

Case history continued

Later that day, the isolate is identified by matrix-assisted laser desorption ionization time-of-flight mass spectrometry (MALDI-TOF) as *Klebsiella pneumoniae*. The initial susceptibility testing suggests this is a possible carbapenemase-producing *Enterobacteriales* (CPE) and antibiotics are changed but he remains acutely septic. The patient goes for a laparotomy and pus is drained from the abdomen from which a similar bacterium to the blood, a carbapenemase-producing *K. pneumoniae*, is isolated. His treatment is changed to colistin and amikacin and he improves over the next 3 days. Subsequently, he is discharged to a general ward and the same isolate is recovered from a rectal swab.

Questions

34.4 What are CPEs?

34.5 How are CPEs best confirmed in the microbiology laboratory?

34.6 What options are available for treatment of this patient's infection?

34.7 How can the spread of CPEs be prevented in hospitals?

34.8 How long should patients remain in isolation while an in-patient?

Answers

34.4 What are CPEs?

These bacteria, first described in the United States in the mid-1990s, produce enzymes that hydrolyse all β-lactam molecules, including the carbapenems. Consequently, there are greatly reduced options for treatment as many of these bacteria are also resistant to other classes of antibiotics such as quinolones and aminoglycosides. There are several categories of CPEs with differing geographical distributions, for example NDM-1 found in the Indian sub-continent (Fig. 34.1), and *K. pneumoniae* carbapenemases (KPC) are found in southern Europe where many belong to one clone, CC258. Other carbapenem-resistant bacteria not mediated by carbapenemases, may be resistant through efflux pumps, porin loss, or AmpC cephalosporinases. These are often referred to as carbapenem-resistant *Enterobacterales* or CRE.

34.5 How are CPEs best confirmed in the microbiology laboratory?

Unlike, for instance methicillin-resistant *Staphylococcus aureus*, where resistance is mediated by a relatively limited number of mechanisms, there are many different mechanisms conferring carbapenem resistance in *Enteroboacteriales* (Fig. 34.1). This makes laboratory detection challenging. The presence of CPEs may initially be suspected by the demonstration of resistance to β-lactam antibiotics and a high minimum inhibitory concentration (MIC) of ertapenem. Other phenotypic tests can confirm and or categorize the mechanism, including the modified Hodge Test and inhibition by chelating agents such as EDTA (indicative of metallo-β-lactamases). MALDI-TOF MS has been used for CPE confirmation but this technology is still largely a research tool for this purpose. Molecular methods include the detection of resistance genes by in-house and commercial PCR, micro-arrays, and whole genome sequencing, but the last 2 are largely confined to research or to reference laboratories. However, this is changing rapidly as the technology becomes cheaper and simpler.

34.6 What options are available for treatment of this patient's infection?

Definitive therapy will depend on the full antimicrobial susceptibility testing. Amongst the options are a fluoroquinolone (often resistant), an aminoglycoside (some isolates remain susceptible to amikacin), colistin (a polymixin that was largely discarded for use some decades back because of toxicity), tigecycline (some isolates are resistant), and fosfomycin (mainly for urinary infection). Newer agents such as ceftazidime-avibactam and aztreonam-avibactam show some promise in selected

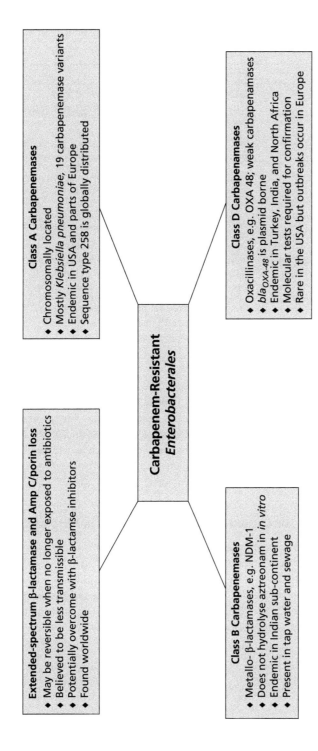

Figure 34.1 The classification of carbapenem-resistant *Enterobacterales*.

Extended-spectrum β-lactamase and Amp C/porin loss
- May be reversible when no longer exposed to antibiotics
- Believed to be less transmissible
- Potentially overcome with β-lactamse inhibitors
- Found worldwide

Class A Carbapenemases
- Chromosomally located
- Mostly *Klebsiella pneumoniae*, 19 carbapenemase variants
- Endemic in USA and parts of Europe
- Sequence type 258 is globally distributed

Carbapenem-Resistant *Enterobacterales*

Class B Carbapenemases
- Metallo-β-lactamases, e.g. NDM-1
- Does not hydrolyse aztreonam in *in vitro*
- Endemic in Indian sub-continent
- Present in tap water and sewage

Class D Carbapenamases
- Oxacillinases, e.g. OXA 48; weak carbapenamases
- *bla*$_{OXA-48}$ is plasmid borne
- Endemic in Turkey, India, and North Africa
- Molecular tests required for confirmation
- Rare in the USA but outbreaks occur in Europe

Table 34.1 Antibiotics for the therapy of carbapenem-resistant Enterobacteriaceal infections

Antibiotic	Comments
Colistin	Takes 2 days for drug concentrations to achieve a steady state; significant risk of nephrotoxicity; usually used in combination
Aminoglycosides	Many isolates are resistant; nephrotoxicity increased in critically ill patients and those on colistin; not used alone
Tigecycline	Bacteriostatic and should be used in combination; high doses associated with reduced mortality rates
Fosfomycin	Main indication is for urinary tract infection; used intravenously as salvage therapy when options limited
Newer agents e.g. ceftazidime-avibactam, aztreonam-avibactam, eravacycline	Some agents show promise, but most have not been fully evaluated in clinical trials. There also gaps such as ceftazidime-avibactam is not active against NDMs.
Carbapenems	Controversial; may be useful in combination for OXA48 infections when carbapenem MIC is low; better activity if administered by continuous infusion

NDM, New Delhi metallo-β-lactamase; MIC, minimum inhibitory concentration.

patients, but further studies are awaited. Despite the detection of genes coding for carbapenemases, high-dose carbapenems may be used (possibly administered by continuous infusion) if the isolate is susceptible on testing and/or the minimum inhibitory concentration is low. Combination therapy such as with amikacin and colistin, or even including 3 agents, is often used as many believe that patients do better (Table 34.1).

34.7 How can the spread of CPEs be prevented in hospitals?

Early recognition of cases, rigorous contact precautions including long-sleeved gowns, patient isolation, and designated nursing are important in preventing spread. At-risk patients should be screened, including this patient who was hospitalized in Asia. Enhanced environmental hygiene is essential as these organisms may persist in the environment. There are no recognized and validated methods for the decolonization of patients with ESBLs and CREs.

34.8 How long should patients remain in isolation while an in-patient?

It is not known. Patients may be colonized for considerable periods of time, if not indefinitely. Weekly rectal screening of positive patients is probably wise while in hospital and all known CPE patients should be isolated for the duration of hospitalization.

Acknowledgements

Thanks to Professor Martin Cormican for reviewing the draft.

Further reading

Hawkey PM, Warren RE, Livermore DM, McNulty C, Enoch DA, et al. Treatment of infections caused by multidrug-resistant Gram-negative bacteria; report of the British Society for Antimicrobial Chemotherapy/Healthcare Infection Society/British Infection Association Joint Working Party. *J Antimicrob Chemother* 2018; **73**: iii2–iii78.

Logan LK, Weinstein RA. The epidemiology of carbapenem-resistant Enterobacteriaceae: the impact and evolution of a global menace. *J Infect Dis* 2017; **215**: S28–36.

Lutgring JD, Limbago BM. The problem of carbapenemase-producing carbapenem-resistant-Enterobacteriaceae detection. *J Clin Microbiol* 2016; **54**: 529–34.

Magiorakos AP, Burns K, Rodríguez Bano J, Borg M, Daikos G, et al. Infection prevention and control measures and tools for the prevention of entry of carbapenem-resistant *Enterobacteriaceae* into healthcare settings: guidance from the European Centre for Disease Prevention and Control. *Antimicrob Resist In* 2017; **6**: 113. doi.10.1186/s13756-017-0259-z.

Murray PR, Masur H. Current approaches to the diagnosis of bacterial and fungal bloodstream infections for the ICU. *Critical Care Med* 2012; **40**: 3277–82.

Case 35

Andrew Woodhouse

Case history

A 27-year-old UK-born man presents to the Emergency Department (ED) with a 2-day history of fever, headache, intermittent diarrhoea, and shaking episodes which sound like rigors. He has recently returned from a trip to Africa where he travelled through a number of countries including South Africa, Kenya, Uganda, and Tanzania over a 4-month period. He has been back in the United Kingdom for 2 weeks. He took daily doxycycline as malaria prophylaxis for the first 6 weeks of his trip but not subsequently. Physical examination confirms fever (39.5 °C) but there are no other abnormal findings.

Questions

35.1 Does malaria need to be considered here?

35.2 Which species of malaria could be a cause in this case?

35.3 What diagnostic tests should be requested to investigate the possibility of malaria?

Answers

35.1 Does malaria need to be considered here?

Yes. He has returned from a malaria-endemic region and even if he had taken prophylaxis appropriately, malaria is among the most important conditions in the differential diagnosis of fever in this setting. The differential diagnosis of his fever is broad and includes other travel-associated infections including enteric fever, dengue, and other arboviruses, hepatitis, leptospirosis, and rickettsial infection. Detail of a traveller's itinerary, activities while away, contacts including sexual contacts are important when considering possible causes of fever. Where did he go, what did he do, and who with are important questions?

35.2 Which species of malaria could be a cause in this case?

There are 5 species of malaria which can infect humans: *P. falciparum, P. vivax, P. malariae, P. ovale*, and *P. knowlesi*. He might have been infected with any of the first 4 species in sub-Saharan Africa but *P. falciparum* is the most likely to cause severe disease. *P. falciparum* usually presents within 3 months of infection and although later presentations can occur, it is rare. Other species may present much later, even more than a year from the time of infection.

35.3 What diagnostic tests should be requested to investigate the possibility of malaria?

An urgent malaria blood test needs to be obtained. Microscopy of thick and thin blood films should be requested. The level of expertise required for this may not always be available, particularly out-of-hours in hospitals that see small numbers of cases of malaria. As an adjunct many hospitals now also use rapid diagnostic tests (RDT) which detect either parasite antigens or enzymes and these tests are incorporated into local malaria-testing algorithms. All can detect *P. falciparum* and some are pan-species tests. They are not a substitute for examination of blood films. An initial negative blood film and antigen test should prompt repeat testing after 12–24 hours. At least 3 tests should be sent within 48 hours as malaria is not excluded on the basis of a single negative test.

Case history continued

The laboratory calls back to confirm that his RDT is positive for *P. falciparum* and his blood film shows malaria parasites which the microscopist thinks is a mixed infection of *P. falciparum* and *P. vivax*. Other blood tests show thrombocytopenia (platelets 85 × 10^9 /L), anaemia (Hb 75 g/L), mild hepatitis, and renal impairment (creatinine 310 μmol/L). He is transferred to the high dependency unit for close monitoring.

Questions

35.4 What other information will you ask the laboratory to provide?

35.5 What are his management priorities and with what should he be treated?

35.6 When should his parasite count be repeated?

35.7 Does he require specific treatment for *P. vivax*?

35.8 One of the intensive care physicians asks whether exchange transfusion is indicated—should this be considered?

Answers

35.4 What other information will you ask the laboratory to provide?

An estimate of the percentage parasitaemia—the proportion of red blood cells containing parasites—is helpful in determining severity of malaria or the likelihood of development of severe malaria. A variety of indicators of severe or complicated malaria is recognized and patients with *P. falciparum* malaria should be evaluated with these in mind (Box 35.1). The presence of any of the features below constitutes complicated or severe malaria. Other species can also on occasion cause severe malaria. Thrombocytopenia is almost universal in malaria and does not in itself indicate severe disease.

35.5 What are his management priorities and with what should he be treated?

The laboratory reports a parasitaemia of 15%. He has severe, complicated *P. falciparum* malaria because of the parasitaemia, anaemia, and renal function. He requires effective antimalarial treatment and careful monitoring. He should be managed in a high-dependency environment with careful attention to his haemodynamic state, glycaemic control, and renal and respiratory function. He urgently needs to start on effective antimalarial treatment which in this case should be given parenterally. Intravenous (IV) artesunate is now widely acknowledged as the drug of choice for treatment of severe malaria with a number of trials showing mortality benefit over

---

Box 35.1 Features of severe *P. falciparum* malaria

- Neurological involvement—seizures, reduced consciousness, confusion
- Renal impairment—oliguria or raised serum creatinine (WHO definition > 265 μmol/L)
- Metabolic acidosis (pH < 7.3)
- Hypoglycaemia (glucose < 2.2 μmol/L)
- Pulmonary oedema
- Hypotension/shock
- Severe anaemia (Hb < 80 g/L)
- Spontaneous bleeding/evidence of disseminated intravascular coagulation
- Haemoglobinuria
- Parasitaemia > 10% (US CDC defines 5%; > 2% increases chance of developing severe disease even if otherwise well)

Adapted with permission from Lalloo DG, Shingadia D, Bell DJ, Beeching NJ, Whitty CJM, et al. (2016). UK malaria treatment guidelines 2016. *J Infect* 72:635–649. DOI: 10.1016/j.jinf.2016.02.001.

---

quinine and should be used where available. He should receive at least 24 hours of IV treatment and provided improvement is demonstrated this can be followed by a full course of oral artemesinin combination therapy such as artemether-lumefantrine. This drug would be appropriate oral treatment for uncomplicated *P. falciparum* infection with alternatives being oral atovaquone-proguanil or quinine plus doxycycline.

If artesunate is not available, treatment should be started with intravenous quinine to avoid delay. Quinine treatment can be continued orally once swallowing is safe but will require the use of a second agent such as doxycycline or clindamycin orally for 7 days after the initial treatment.

35.6 When should his parasite count be repeated?

Monitoring parasitaemia is recommended to check for clearance and response to treatment but the count may not drop significantly in the first 24 hours or so. Repeat blood films for parasitaemia every 24 hours is a reasonable frequency for the first 2–3 days.

35.7 Does he require specific treatment for *P. vivax*?

Not initially. If he does have mixed infection, the treatment he receives acutely will treat both *P. falciparum* and *P. vivax*. If *P. vivax* is confirmed by blood film, he will require a course of primaquine to eradicate the hypnozoite phase of the parasite to prevent recrudescent disease later.

35.8 One of the intensive care physicians asks whether exchange transfusion is indicated—should this be considered?

In the past, exchange transfusion had been recommended for extreme parasitaemia and severe malaria although it was not a universally accepted treatment. Based on current evidence it is no longer recommended and modern guidelines reflect this.

Further reading

CDC. Malaria diagnosis and treatment in the United States. 2015. https://www.cdc.gov/malaria/diagnosis_treatment/

Lalloo DG, Shigadia D, Bell DJ, Beeching NJ, Whitty CJM, et al. UK malaria treatment guidelines 2016. *J Infect* 2016; 72: 635–49.

Severe malaria. *Trop Med Int Health* 2014; 19: 7–131.

Sinclair D, Donegan S, Isba R, Lalloo DG. Artesunate versus quinine for treating severe malaria. *Cochrane Database Syst Rev* 2012; **6**. CD005967.

White NJ, Pukrittayakamee S, Hien TT, Faiz MA, Mokuolu OA, et al. Malaria. *Lancet* 2014; 383: 723–35.

Case 36

Andrew Woodhouse

Case history

A 55-year-old woman is referred to hospital with fever, headache, and a maculopapular rash. She has been unwell for about 2 weeks, having initially developed a sore throat for which she received a course of amoxicillin with minimal response. Fever has been a feature throughout her illness but the rash and headache developed after 4–5 days of illness. There is no history of recent travel and she is usually well and on no medication. On examination her throat is inflamed but her tonsils are not enlarged. She has a number of shallow ulcers on her tongue and small non-tender palpable cervical lymph nodes bilaterally. There is a maculopapular rash involving her upper trunk and also her face. A number of tests including human immunodeficiency virus (HIV) serology are requested.

Her HIV test is positive with p24 antigen and anti-HIV antibody detected, confirmed on repeat testing and she also has mildly deranged liver enzymes with a raised alanine aminotransferase (ALT). An HIV viral load is over 100,000 copies/ml of plasma. A CD4 lymphocyte count is 280 cells/mm^3.

Questions

36.1 What is a differential for her presentation and, in addition to HIV testing, what investigations should be included in her initial work-up?

36.2 How long is she likely to have been infected with HIV?

36.3 What are the clinical manifestations of acute HIV infection?

36.4 Is antiretroviral treatment indicated in the setting of acute HIV infection?

Answers

36.1 What is a differential for her presentation and, in addition to HIV testing, what investigations should be included in her initial work-up?

Her presentation is consistent with a mononucleosis-type illness with fever, sore throat, and lymphadenopathy. The differential is wide but includes acute infection with Epstein–Barr virus (EBV), cytomegalovirus (CMV), toxoplasmosis, syphilis, and HIV. Testing for these infections should be requested along with routine haematology and biochemistry investigations.

36.2 How long is she likely to have been infected with HIV?

The clinical presentation is consistent with an acute HIV seroconversion illness suggesting infection has been acquired recently, probably within the last 2–6 weeks.

36.3 What are the clinical manifestations of acute HIV infection?

The clinical features of acute HIV infection are variable but up to 50% of infected individuals will have some combination of symptoms. The non-specific nature of the symptoms means that the diagnosis is not considered and many people are not tested for HIV infection at the time of their presentation with acute illness. Oral ulceration and rash are particularly suggestive and would be unusual in EBV infection, for instance. Table 36.1 outlines some of the clinical and laboratory features of acute

Table 36.1 Clinical and laboratory manifestations of acute HIV infection

Feature	Approx. frequency
Fever	> 90%
Lymphadenopathy	70%
Rash	70%
Sore throat	80%
Myalgia/arthralgia	50%
Headache	40%
Transaminitis	20%
Leucopaenia	40%

Source: data from de Jong MD, Hulsebosch HJ and Lange JM. (1991). Clinical, virological and immunological features of primary HIV-1 infection. *Genitourin Med* 67(5): 367–373.

HIV infection and highlights the non-specific nature of the illness. A high index of suspicion for the possibility of HIV infection should be maintained and a low threshold for testing applied after appropriate discussion with patients presenting with a compatible illness.

Although there is a window period following HIV infection when antibodies are not detectable, newer-generation diagnostic tests are likely to detect antibody as early as 3 weeks after infection. Simultaneous detection of p24 viral antigen is also a component of these sensitive combination assays and should be used if acute infection is suspected. Direct detection of virus by PCR is even more sensitive and can be used diagnostically but also to quantify the viral load which is typically very high during the acute illness, making patients highly infectious.

36.4 Is antiretroviral treatment indicated in the setting of acute HIV infection?

Yes. There has been a shift in recommendations regarding when to start antiretroviral treatment in HIV infection in recent years. Despite highly effective and tolerable treatment combinations, HIV cannot be eradicated even when treatment is given soon after infection. Patients recover spontaneously from acute infection, and as they generate an HIV-specific immune response they will reduce their viral load and recover CD4 cell numbers which are often suppressed during acute infection. A conventional approach for many years was to monitor patients' immune function by CD4 lymphocyte count and to introduce antiretroviral therapy when CD4 counts fell to levels around 350 cells/mm³. A number of studies showing improved outcomes and preservation of immune function when antiviral treatment is not delayed based on CD4 count, however, have informed recent guidelines. Most now support the introduction of antiviral treatment as soon as HIV infection is diagnosed, irrespective of symptoms or immune parameters. Patient acceptance and willingness to embark on treatment, which is likely to be indefinite, is a critical requirement.

Most authorities would now recommend the introduction of treatment soon after a diagnosis of acute HIV infection. There may be benefits in terms of subsequent immune control of virus by treating early in infection and limiting the extent of development of the viral reservoir.

Case history continued

The patient does not use intravenous drugs and has been with the same sexual partner for 2 years. Her partner is unaware of his HIV status but is tested and is HIV-antibody positive. He has a CD4 count of 80 cells/mm³ and an HIV viral load of 32,000 copies/ml of plasma. He feels well and is on no regular medications but 5 years ago had an episode of shingles and was admitted to hospital 3 years ago with pneumococcal pneumonia.

Questions

36.5   How long is he likely to have been infected with HIV?

36.6   Is he at risk of developing complications of HIV infection?

36.7   What treatment approach should be adopted in his situation?

Answers

36.5 How long is he likely to have been infected with HIV?

Although he has not been aware of his HIV infection he is severely immunocompromised, as indicated by his very low CD4 lymphocyte count. Although some individuals can progress rapidly to severe immunodeficiency following infection, it is likely that he has been infected for years. Reactivation of herpes zoster causing shingles is common in patients with HIV and is a clue to infection. Similarly, pneumococcal pneumonia and invasive pneumococcal disease should be viewed as an indicator of possible underlying HIV infection and should prompt testing.

36.6 Is he at risk of developing complications of HIV infection?

Yes. He is at high risk of complications of HIV due to his low CD4 count. The risk of opportunistic infections and malignancies increase with falling CD4 lymphocyte count. His CD4 count puts him at risk of *Pneumocystis jirovecii* pneumonia (PCP), toxoplasmosis (if toxoplasma seropositive), and disseminated *Mycobacterium avium* complex (MAC). Table 36.2 indicates the risk of important selected opportunistic infection relative to CD4 count.

36.7 What treatment approach should be adopted in his situation?

The therapeutic approach is twofold. He needs antiretroviral treatment in order to suppress viral replication and allow CD4 lymphocyte recovery. In addition, selected antimicrobial prophylaxis to prevent development of opportunistic infections should be started. Co-trimoxazole is effective at preventing PCP and also toxoplasma reactivation. Primary prophylaxis for MAC is usually started at CD4 counts

Table 36.2 Opportunistic infection risk in HIV relative to CD4 lymphocyte count

Opportunistic infection	CD4 lymphocyte count
Tuberculosis	Risk at all CD4 counts
Pneumocystis jirovecii	< 200 cells/mm³
Toxoplasmosis	< 100 cells/mm³
Mycobacterium avium complex	< 100 cells/mm³
Cytomegalovirus retinitis	< 50 cells/mm³
Cryptococcal meningoencephalitis	< 50 cells/mm³

below 50 cells/mm³ but some clinicians would consider giving azithromycin in this situation. Prophylaxis is continued until CD4 lymphocytes show sustained recovery to above the levels of risk and can then be stopped. Antiretroviral therapy remains the most important intervention in preventing opportunistic infections and restoring health to patients with HIV infection.

Further reading

BHIVA guidelines for the treatment of HIV-1-positive adults with antiretroviral therapy 2015 (2016 interim update). Available at: https://www.bhiva.org/HIV-1-treatment-guidelines.aspx.

Braun DL, Kouyos RD, Balmer B, Grube C, Weber R, et al. Frequency and spectrum of unexpected clinical manifestations of primary HIV-1 infection. *Clin Infect Dis* 2015; **61:** 1013–21. Epub 2015 May 19.

De Jong MD, Hulsebosch HJ, Lange MA. Clinical, virological and immunological features of primary HIV-1 infection. *Genitourin Med* 1991; **67:** 367–73.

INSIGHT START Study Group, Lundgren JD, Babiker AG, et al. Initiation of antiretroviral therapy in early asymptomatic HIV infection. *N Engl J Med* 2015; **373:** 795–807.

Maartens G, Celum C, Lewin SR. HIV infection: epidemiology, pathogenesis, treatment, and prevention. *Lancet* 2014; **384:** 258–71.

Case 37

Andrew Woodhouse

Case history

A 23-year old soldier presents with a non-tender ulcerated lesion on his distal right forearm (Fig. 37.1) with nodules extending proximally up his arm and a palpable lymph node in his right axilla. He returned from a period of jungle training in Belize 8 weeks previously. He is systemically well.

Questions

37.1 What conditions should be considered here?

37.2 What is the most likely diagnosis and how can the diagnosis be proven?

Answers

37.1 What conditions should be considered here?

The nodular ulcerating skin lesion raises the possibility of cutaneous leishmaniasis but other uncommon infections including non-tuberculous *Mycobacteria* spp., and fungal infections such as cutaneous sporotrichosis or blastomycosis need consideration. When considering ulcerating nodular skin lesions in general, non-infective pathologies need to be borne in mind and depending on the presentation might include conditions such as pyoderma gangrenosum, prurigo nodularis, cutaneous sarcoidosis, and malignant diseases including primary cutaneous malignancies and lymphoma.

37.2 What is the most likely diagnosis and how can the diagnosis be proven?

Based on the history and appearance (Fig. 37.1), this is likely to be cutaneous leishmaniasis (CL) acquired during his training in Latin America. Confirmation of CL is best done using material from a punch or wedge biopsy taken from the edge of the lesion.

Biopsy material should first be used to produce 'touch preparations' on a glass slide for microscopy using Giemsa or Leishman's stain. The hallmark of diagnosis by direct visualization is the identification of intracellular amastigotes within macrophages, which are distinguished by the presence of a nucleus and a kinetoplast.

Biopsy material should then be sent for histopathology, polymerase chain reaction (PCR) tests, and culture (if available). Histopathology may similarly demonstrate

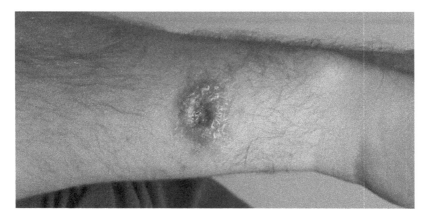

Figure 37.1 Ulcerated forearm lesion (see colour plate).

Reproduced courtesy of Lt Col (Prof) Mark Bailey, Consultant Physician and Professor in Infectious Diseases and Tropical Medicine, Birmingham Heartlands Hospital, Warwick Medical School, and Royal Centre for Defence Medicine, UK.

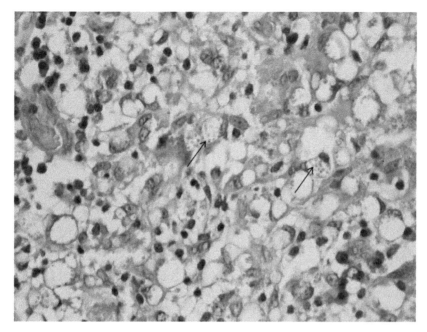

Figure 37.2 Intracellular amastigotes (arrow) are present in the cytoplasm of the histiocytes. H&E ×600 (see colour plate).

Reproduced courtesy of University Hospitals Birmingham NHS Foundation Trust, UK.

amastigotes (Fig. 37.2) although the yield from histology is lower in older lesions and secondarily infected ulcers may show predominantly non-specific inflammation.

PCR tests are the most sensitive method of laboratory diagnosis and can also identify the *Leishmania* species involved.

Culture using Novy–McNeal–Nicolle (NNN) medium is becoming less common and has a low yield overall.

Questions

37.3 What species of leishmania is most likely to be the cause in this case.

37.4 Depending on the species are there any particular complications that need to be considered?

37.5 What treatment options can be considered in this case if testing confirms *L.(V.) braziliensis*?

37.6 What monitoring is required for patients treated with intravenous stibogluconate?

Answers

37.3 What species of leishmania is most likely to be the cause in this case

This is so-called New World CL, having been acquired in Latin America. Parasites of the *Leishmania (Vianna) braziliensis* and *Leishmania (L) mexicana* complexes could both be responsible in a returnee from Belize. PCR tests can provide information on the species.

37.4 Depending on the species are there any particular complications that need to be considered?

L.(V.) braziliensis is known to cause mucosal leishmaniasis (ML), which is a destructive process involving the oral and nasal mucosa and which can develop from primary infection elsewhere and be quite distant from the face. It is usually caused by *L.(V.) braziliensis* infection acquired in Latin America, but very few cases have been described from Belize and other countries north of Costa Rica. Nonetheless in cases of *L.(V) braziliensis*, a careful review of symptoms and examination by nasoendoscopy of the oropharynx including the vocal cords should be considered with biopsy of any abnormal looking tissue to exclude ML.

37.5 What treatment options can be considered in this case if testing confirms *L.(V.) braziliensis*?

Options for the treatment of CL include local therapy and oral or parenteral systemic treatment. The traditional recommendation for treatment of CL caused by *L.(V.) braziliensis* is with parenteral pentavalent antimony compounds (e.g. sodium stibogluconate). The rationale for systemic treatment is to avoid progression to ML. This is in contrast to treatment of Old World CL where spontaneous resolution occurs over time or where there is a good response to local injections of stibogluconate. Intra-lesional stibogluconate is recommended for uncomplicated CL where the ulcer is relatively small and not caused by *L.(V.) braziliensis*, when systemic treatment is required. A number of oral systemic agents have been used to treat CL including the imidazole antifungals, but with inconsistent results. More recently miltefosine, an oral alkylphosphocholine which interferes with cell signalling pathways in the parasite membrane, has become available. Miltefosine is approved for the treatment of cutaneous and mucocutaneous leishmaniasis due to *L.(V.) braziliensis* and would be a treatment option in this case. There are less data on its use in other species, particularly the Old World forms of CL, but experience is accumulating.

37.6 What monitoring is required for patients treated with intravenous stibogluconate?

The pentavalent antimony compounds can cause anaemia, hepatitis, pancreatitis, and non-specific ST segment changes on electrocardiogram (ECG). Overall they are tolerated reasonably well in younger and smaller patients. Weekly blood test monitoring of FBC, urea and electrolytes, liver function tests, and amylase, and a weekly ECG should be undertaken.

Further reading

Bailey MS, Lockwood DN. Cutaneous leishmaniasis. *Clin Dermatol* 2007; 25: 203–11.

Blum J, Buffet P, Visser L, Harms G, Bailey MS, et al. LeishMan recommendations for treatment of cutaneous and mucosal leishmaniasis in travellers. *J Travel Med* 2014; 21: 116–29.

Burza S, Croft SL, Boelaert M. Leishmaniasis. *Lancet* 2018; 392: 951–90.

Copeland NK, Aronson NE. Leishmaniasis: treatment updates and clinical practice guidelines review. *Curr Opin Infect Dis* 2015; 28: 426–37.

Hodiamont CJ, Kager PA, Bart A, de Vries HJ, van Thiel PP, et al. Species directed therapy for leishmaniasis in returning travellers: a comprehensive guide. *PLoS Negl Trop Dis* 2014; 8: e2832.

Case 38

Andrew Woodhouse

Case history

A 46-year-old kidney transplant recipient presents with a 2-week history of sore throat, sweats, and fever 11 months after he received a cadaveric renal transplant. His transplant has been successful with no significant post-operative complications to date. He was cytomegalovirus (CMV), Epstein-Barr virus (EBV), and toxoplasma antibody-positive prior to transplant and received a CMV-negative organ, that is, CMV D–/R+. He received oral valganciclovir 900 mg daily for the first 3 months following transplantation as CMV prophylaxis. His immunosuppression is prednisolone, ciclosporin, and mycophenolate, and he has good graft function with a normal creatinine. On examination he is found to have enlarged non-inflamed tonsils, small-volume cervical lymph nodes, and his liver edge is palpable and slightly tender. Initial blood tests show a lymphocytosis and mildly raised transaminases. A plasma CMV viral load is < 300 copies/ml.

Questions

38.1 What are the possible causes of his fever?

38.2 What additional investigations may be helpful in determining the cause of his illness?

Answers

38.1 What are the possible causes of his fever?

Evaluating fever in immunocompromised hosts requires consideration of a range of typical and opportunistic pathogens in addition to non-infectious causes. He is now 11 months' post-transplant but remains significantly immunosuppressed. He received valganciclovir post-operatively for 3 months as prophylaxis because of his CMV seropositive status. Late reactivation of CMV should always be considered after prophylaxis stops but he is not at high risk. The absence of detectable systemic virus makes CMV disease unlikely. His sore throat, fever, and lymphadenopathy raises the possibility of pharyngitis due either to bacteria or viruses. He also has features of a mononucleosis-type illness with a mild hepatitis and the differential in an immunocompetent host would include primary EBV or toxoplasma infection. His pre-transplant serology indicates previous infection with both pathogens. Reactivation of toxoplasmosis in the context of solid organ transplantation typically causes focal disease in the brain or elsewhere but EBV reactivation can occur and mimic an infectious mononucleosis-type illness. This forms part of a spectrum of conditions known collectively as post-transplant lymphoproliferative disorders (PTLD). Primary HIV infection must not be forgotten as a cause of mononucleosis type illness and should be excluded (see Case 36). His graft function is excellent so rejection is unlikely.

38.2 What additional investigations may be helpful in determining the cause of his illness?

Throat swabs for bacterial culture and viral polymerase chain reaction (PCR) will help to exclude a conventional cause for his presentation. An HIV test should be done using a combined antibody/antigen test to exclude early infection. In the context of a mononucleosis-type illness and known EBV seropositivity, PTLD is a definite possibility and an EBV viral load should be requested. EBV serology alone is not generally helpful in the diagnosis of PTLD and may be misleading, even in acute EBV infection following transplantation due to immunosuppression abrogating the immune response. With the possibility of PTLD in mind, a computerized tomography (CT) scan of neck, chest, abdomen, and pelvis should be undertaken to identify any areas of focal disease that may be amenable to biopsy. Although PTLD represents a lymphoproliferative disorder, lymph node involvement is not a universal feature and many patients may have no obvious involvement of peripheral lymph nodes detectable on clinical examination. Focal disease in the form of pulmonary nodules or lesions in the liver, spleen, or small bowel may be seen on CT and help to direct biopsy. Positron emission tomography scanning with CT (PET-CT, Positron Emission Tomography-Computerized Tomography) may increase the sensitivity of imaging by detecting smaller foci of abnormal lymphoid tissue and abnormal bone marrow.

Patients with PTLD can present at any time after transplant, often within the first year but timing will vary depending on pre-transplant EBV status.

Case history continued

His swabs are negative for bacteria and viruses as is his HIV test. His plasma EBV viral load is 25,000 copies/ml. Atypical lymphocytes are seen in peripheral blood and his lymphocyte count is rising. The CT scan identifies enlarged intra-abdominal lymph nodes in the coeliac axis and retroperitoneal area with evidence of small bowel thickening in the ileum.

A laparoscopic biopsy is undertaken and lymph node tissue is obtained for histology.

Questions

38.3 How can PTLD be confirmed?

38.4 What are the treatment approaches to consider in PTLD?

38.5 Is there a role for EBV viral load monitoring after transplantation?

Answers

38.3 How can PTLD be confirmed?

A diagnosis of PTLD should be based on histology which requires biopsy of involved tissue. An excisional biopsy is preferred to a needle biopsy. Preferably, the sample should be examined by a pathologist with experience in the diagnosis of PTLD. The World Health Organization has developed a classification system with 4 categories. These categories are:

1. Non-destructive PTLD
2. Polymorphic PTLD
3. Monomorphic PTLD
4. Classical Hodgkin's lymphoma PTLD

38.4 What are the treatment approaches to consider in PTLD?

The main initial approach to PTLD is a carefully monitored reduction of immuno-suppression (ROI). The aim is to allow recovery of the patient's immune system resulting in expansion of EBV specific cytotoxic T-cells that can help control the EBV–driven proliferation of B lymphocytes. In addition, the use of B cell-targeted antibody therapy with the monoclonal rituximab (anti-CD20) has become a standard approach with good response rates in post-transplant PTLD. In patients not responding to ROI and rituximab, cytotoxic chemotherapy will generally be used, typically a cyclophosphamide based regimen. Although antiviral therapy with ganciclovir or aciclovir is often used adjunctively there is little robust evidence to support this practice which is largely based on historic, anecdotal reports of benefit.

38.5 Is there a role for EBV viral load monitoring after transplantation?

Monitoring of EBV viral load can be useful as an adjunct in monitoring response to treatment of PTLD. Routine EBV viral load monitoring following transplant-ation is fairly routine following haemopoietic stem cell transplants and increasingly common after solid organ transplant (SOT). There are some uncertainties with this approach, in part due to difficulties with interpretation of the viral load. Many sero-positive patients will have detectable virus in plasma or peripheral blood mono-nuclear cells but will not progress to development of PTLD. A rising viral load over time is more predictive of the development of PTLD than a stable detectable level. Viral load monitoring in high-risk SOT situations such as a seronegative recipient of an EBV seropositive graft may have more merit. Many transplant centres will intervene by ROI in the context of a rising viral load although the threshold for such intervention has not been precisely defined. Use of rituximab in a pre-emptive manner has also been considered if ROI does not lead to reductions in viral load but there is insufficient evidence to date to be able to make firm recommendations.

Further reading

Green M, Michaels MG. Epstein–Barr virus infection and post transplant lymphoproliferative disorder. *Am J Transplantation* 2013; **13**: 41–54.

Parker A, Bowles K, Bradley JA, Emery V, Featherstone C, et al. on behalf of the Haemato-Oncology Task Force of the British Committee for Standards in Haematology and British Transplantation Society. Management of post-transplant lymphoproliferative disorder in adult solid organ transplant recipients—BCSH and BTS Guidelines. *Br J Haematol* 2010; **149**: 693–705.

San-Juan R, Comoli P, Caillard S, Moulin B, Hirsch HH, et al. On behalf of the ESCMID Study Group of Infection in Compromised Hosts (ESGICH). Epstein–Barr virus related post-transplant lymphoproliferative disorder in solid organ transplant recipients. *Clin Microbiol Infect* 2014; **20**: 109–18.

Swerdlow SH, Campo E, Pileri SA, Harris NL, Stein H, et al. The 2016 revision of the World Health Organization classification of lymphoidneoplasms. *Blood* 2016; **127**: 2375–90.

Section 7

Infections in pregnancy and the neonate

Case 39

Katie Jeffery

Case history

A 32-year-old schoolteacher presents to her General Practitioner (GP) concerned that she has been exposed to a child in the classroom with a rash illness that she has been told is due to Parvovirus B19, although this is unconfirmed. She is 15-weeks pregnant.

Questions

39.1 What further history should be taken?

39.2 What viral infections commonly causing a rash illness are of particular concern in pregnancy and why?

39.3 What testing should be considered in this case?

39.4 Should she be excluded from work?

Answers

39.1 What further history should be taken?

An immunization and previous exposure history

This is especially important for individuals not born in the United Kingdom, as vaccination coverage can vary. The history should include measles, mumps, and rubella (MMR) immunization. If the rash she was exposed to had been suspected varicella-zoster virus (VZV), a history of chickenpox, or VZV immunization in the patient should also be checked. Although VZV seroprevalence is 95% in UK-born women, in those born in less temperate climates this may be significantly lower, for example in Sri Lanka it is as low as 50% in women of child-bearing age, therefore ethnicity is an important consideration. If the patient has a clear history of chickenpox or shingles prior to becoming pregnant, she can be reassured. If there is no history of prior VZV infection or immunization, she should be tested urgently for the presence of VZV immunoglobulin G (IgG). If IgG-negative, consult Public Health England guidelines. VZV immunoglobulin or aciclovir should be considered, depending on the date and nature of the exposure and the gestation.

What were the dates and nature of the contact with the child who was unwell?

The infectious phase of Parvovirus B19 is up to 10 days prior to rash onset until 1 day after the rash appears. Significant contact for viruses spread by the respiratory route is defined as face-to-face contact or 15 minutes within the same room.

Does she currently have any symptoms?

For example, fever, rash, arthralgias, headache, respiratory symptoms, inflammation of the eyes.

39.2 What viral infections commonly causing a rash illness are of particular concern in pregnancy and why?

Parvovirus B19

If infection occurs at less than 20 weeks gestation there is a 9% excess foetal loss (risk 15% vs 5% in control group) and a 3% risk of hydrops foetalis. If this occurs there is about 50% foetal mortality. There is no evidence of Parvovirus B19-associated teratogenicity.

Rubella

At less than 11 weeks gestation there is a 90% risk of major congenital abnormalities including sensori-neural deafness, retinopathy, cataract, microphthalmia, and congenital heart disease. At 11–16 weeks gestation the risk decreases to 20%. From 16–20 weeks there is a small risk of deafness only. Above 20 weeks gestation there is no increased risk of foetal abnormalities.

Measles

There is an increased rate of foetal loss and premature delivery. There is no evidence to support a risk of congenital abnormalities.

Varicella-zoster virus

Congenital varicella syndrome includes low birth weight, neurological involvement, eye and skeletal abnormalities, skin scarring, and limb hypoplasia. At less than 13 weeks gestation the risk is 0.4%. At 13–20 weeks it is around 2%. Rarely, congenital varicella syndrome has been reported in pregnancies up to 28 weeks.

Neonates may develop disseminated haemorrhagic chickenpox if exposed between 4 days prior to and 2 days post-delivery, with increased risk of death.

Zika

An expert panel convened by the World Health Organization (WHO) in 2016 concluded, from the available evidence (outbreaks of Zika virus infection and clusters of microcephaly), that Zika virus infection during pregnancy is a cause of congenital brain abnormalities, including microcephaly.

39.3 What testing should be considered in this case?

Parvovirus B19 infection may be asymptomatic, and therefore it is important to test for Parvovirus B19 infection in all cases of possible/probable exposure in this setting. Serum should be tested for both B19 IgG and IgM. Approximately 50% of the UK young adult population will be immune to Parvovirus B19 infection (IgG detected, IgM not detected) and can be reassured. If no IgG or IgM are detected, the woman should be re-tested one month after her last exposure.

Testing for measles virus immune status should be considered, in individuals with no or incomplete immunization history.

Testing for rubella immunity is indicated in individuals with no or incomplete immunization history. Serum should be tested for Rubella IgG and IgM, and testing should be repeated 4 weeks later if the patient is shown to be susceptible.

If a pregnant woman has had a significant contact with varicella-zoster but has no history of previous VZV or immunization, she should be urgently tested for VZV IgG.

39.4 Should she be excluded from work?

The risk of acquiring Parvovirus B19 infection in the workplace is the same as that in the community or at home, and routine exclusion of susceptible teachers who are less than 21 weeks pregnant is not generally advised. However, if there is an outbreak within the school, consideration could be given to excluding the staff member until 20 weeks gestation.

Case history continued

She has a history of two MMR immunizations and contact with chickenpox virus was not suspected, therefore testing is limited to Parvovirus B19 infection. Her serology results show detectable Parvovirus B19 IgG and IgM, strongly suggesting recent parvovirus infection.

Question

39.5   How should the laboratory confirm Parvovirus B19 infection?

Answer

39.5 How should the laboratory confirm Parvovirus B19 infection?

By two approaches:

1. Test a booking sample if available; if the booking sample is IgG negative, therefore demonstrating seroconversion, primary infection is confirmed.

2. Test a current blood sample for Parvovirus B19 DNA. This may be performed at a reference laboratory, together with confirmation of the IgM result.

Case history continued

Her booking bloods obtained at 9 weeks gestation are negative for B19 IgG and IgM. The reference laboratory has found a Parvovirus DNA level of 5.6×10^6 IU/ml in her most recent sample.

Questions

39.6 How should she be managed at this stage?

39.7 What counselling and advice should she be given on confirmation of Parvovirus B19 in pregnancy?

Answers

39.6 How should she be managed at this stage?

The management of confirmed Parvovirus B19 in pregnancy has become more proactive with the demonstration that foetal blood transfusion improves outcome in hydrops foetalis with a reduction in foetal death. Therefore this woman should be referred for serial ultrasound scanning and Doppler assessment to detect foetal anaemia, heart failure, and hydrops. Scanning should start around 4 weeks after the estimated seroconversion. Referral to a specialist foetal medicine unit is recommended if hydrops is suspected or confirmed.

39.7 What counselling and advice should she be given on confirmation of Parvovirus B19 in pregnancy?

The most likely outcome is a normal pregnancy and birth. There is an increased risk of foetal loss of up to 10%, and a low risk of developing hydrops (around 3%). If the baby does develop hydrops, this may be transient and resolve spontaneously, or effective specialist treatment may be available.

She should avoid contact with other pregnant women until known to be non-infectious—infectious period 7–10 days before the rash (if any) until 1 day after the rash appears. In the absence of rash, it is reasonable to assume the patient is non-infectious if more than 10 days since diagnosis.

Further reading

Carruthers J, Holmes A, Majeed A. A suspected viral rash in pregnancy. *Br Med J* 2017; **356**: 370–1.

Crowcroft NS, Roth CE, Cohen BJ, Miller E. Guidance for control of parvovirus B19 infection in healthcare settings and the community. *J Public Health Med* 1999; **21**: 439–46.

Health Protection Agency. Guidance on the investigation, diagnosis and management of viral illness, or exposure to viral rash illness, in pregnancy. Public Health England 2019.

NICE Clinical Knowledge Summaries: Parvovirus B19 February 2017.

Public Health England (2015). Investigation of Pregnant Women Exposed to Non-Vesicular Rash. UK Standards for Microbiology Investigations. V 30 issue

Public Health England. Immunisation against infectious disease 'The Green Book'.

Case 40

Seilesh Kadambari

Case history

A 12-day-old neonate is brought to the Emergency Department (ED) by his parents with a 1-day history of appearing increasingly drowsy and reduced feeding. The mother reports that she had a normal vaginal delivery and that her membranes ruptured spontaneously 12 hours before delivery. In the ED, the baby is febrile (38.7°C) and tachycardic (heart rate 184). On examination, he is listless. Blood tests reveal a normal full blood count (FBC) and slightly elevated C-reactive protein (CRP) level (18 mg/L) but markedly elevated transaminitis (aspartate transaminase, 2879 U/L [normal range, 15–35 U/L]; alanine transaminase, 1108 U/L [normal range, 13–45 U/L]), and deranged clotting. The neonate is started on empiric antibiotic therapy but the ED doctor also considers a diagnosis of neonatal herpes simplex virus (HSV) disease.

Questions

40.1 What are the potential sources of HSV infection?

40.2 Does this baby have neonatal HSV disease?

40.3 What laboratory tests should be performed to confirm HSV infection?

40.4 What treatment should be started?

40.5 Is further 'suppressive' therapy required?

Answers

40.1 What are the potential sources of HSV infection?

Neonatal HSV infections are most commonly caused by HSV-2 acquired from an infected maternal genital tract. However, HSV-1 is being increasingly identified as causing more genital and neonatal herpes in Europe and in the United States. Almost two-thirds of women who acquire primary genital herpes during pregnancy will be asymptomatic or have non-specific symptoms. Approximately 75% of women with a prior history of genital herpes will have at least 1 recurrence during pregnancy and 14% will have lesions at the time of delivery. Maternal primary infection at the time delivery has the highest risk of transmission (25–57%) compared with recurrent maternal genital HSV (2%). The Royal College of Obstetricians and Gynaecologists (RCOG) recommends caesarean delivery only with primary genital herpes infection with lesions within 6 weeks of delivery. Non-maternal sources account for approximately 5–10% of all cases of neonatal HSV. Box 40.1 outlines the commonest risk factors for neonatal HSV disease.

40.2 Does this baby have neonatal HSV disease?

This neonate has many features which are consistent with disseminated HSV disease. This should be suspected in septic infants who present in the second week of life, even in the absence of vesicular lesions. Fifty per cent of babies with neonatal HSV infection do not have skin or mucous membrane evidence of infection. Furthermore, the neonate has raised transaminases and coagulopathy which are common biochemical findings in disseminated HSV infection. Samples should be obtained before starting antiviral treatment to confirm HSV (but should not delay

---

Box 40.1 Risk factors for transmission of HSV to the neonate

1. Maternal primary infection
2. Lack or low titre of maternal antibody
3. Increasing duration of rupture of membranes
4. Breaching of mucocutaneous barriers (e.g. the use of scalp electrodes)
5. Mode of delivery (vaginal versus caesarean) in women with active shedding of HSV at delivery

Source: data from Pinninti, SG and Kimberlin, DW (2014). Management of neonatal herpes simplex virus infection and exposure. *Arch Dis Child Fetal Neonatal Ed*. 99(3):F240–4. DOI: 10.1136/archdischild-2013-303762.

Table 40.1 Characteristics of the three main presentations of neonatal HSV

Type of disease	Skin, eyes, and mouth (SEM)	Central nervous system (CNS)	Disseminated
Frequency	45%	30%	25%
Symptoms	Vesicles in skin, mouth and conjunctivitis	Skin lesions, fever, lethargy, seizures, abnormal MRI	Skin lesions, sepsis-like syndrome, hepatitis, coagulaopathy, encephalitis
Neurodevelopmental delay	1–5%	70%	27%
Mortality at 1 year	< 1%	4%	29%

Source: data from Pinninti, SG and Kimberlin, DW (2014). Management of neonatal herpes simplex virus infection and exposure. *Arch Dis Child Fetal Neonatal Ed.* 99(3):F240–4. DOI: 10.1136/archdischild-2013-303762.

starting therapy). Table 40.1 describes the commonest clinical characteristics of the 3 main presentations of neonatal HSV.

40.3 What laboratory tests should be performed to confirm HSV infection?

Polymerase chain reaction (PCR) is the diagnostic tool of choice in identifying HSV. Swabs for PCR should be taken from the conjunctiva, mouth, nasopharynx, and anus ('surface swabs'). Vesicular lesions, if present, should be unroofed and tested. PCR is a sensitive tool in detecting HSV in the cerebrospinal fluid (CSF), however, a negative CSF PCR result does not rule out central nervous system (CNS) disease as this could be due to a low viral load or very early disease. Whole-blood PCR may be of benefit in diagnosing HSV disease but cannot be used to determine the extent of the disease or to inform treatment duration.

40.4 What treatment should be started?

All neonates with suspected HSV infection should be treated with IV acyclovir (60 mg/kg/d in 3 divided doses). Babies with disseminated and CNS disease should be treated for 21 days and infants with SEM disease for 14 days. This therapy may be stopped if subsequent investigation rules out a diagnosis of HSV infection.

Neonates with CNS disease should have a repeat lumbar puncture near the end of treatment. Aciclovir should be continued until a negative CSF PCR result is obtained as neonates with positive CSF PCR results at the end of intravenous treatment have been shown to have worse outcomes.

40.5 Is further 'suppressive' therapy required?

A phase III placebo controlled trial showed that infants who received 6 months of oral aciclovir after completing a course of IV aciclovir had improved neuro developmental outcomes and fewer cutaneous recurrences compared to those who received placebo. Recommendations from this are that infants with HSV disease should be treated with 6 months of oral aciclovir (300 mg/m²/dose TDS) after completing intravenous aciclovir. During suppressive therapy, neutrophil counts should be taken regularly (2 weeks, 4 weeks, and then monthly during treatment). Neutropaenia is often transient and can occur during prolonged course of aciclovir. Dose reduction, administration of granulocyte colony-stimulating factor or discontinuation of treatment should be considered in cases with prolonged neutropaenia $< 0.5 \times 10^9$/L.

Further reading

Kimberlin DW, Baley J. Committee on Infectious Diseases; Committee on Fetus and Newborn Guidance on management of asymptomatic neonates born to women with active genital herpes lesions. *Pediatrics* 2013; **131**: 383–6.

Kimberlin DW, Lin CY, Jacobs RF, Powell DA, Corel L, et al. Safety and efficacy of high-dose intravenous acyclovir in the management of neonatal herpes simplex virus infections. *Pediatrics* 2001; **108**: 230–8.

Kimberlin DW, Whitley RJ, Wan W. Oral acyclovir suppression and neurodevelopment after neonatal herpes. *N Engl J Med* 2011; **365**: 1284–92.

Looker KJ, Magaret AS, May MT, Turner KME, Vickerman P, et al. First estimates of the global and regional incidence of neonatal herpes infection. *Lancet Glob Health* 2017; **5**: e300–e309.

Pinninti SG, Kimberlin DW. Management of neonatal herpes simplex virus infection and exposure. *Arch Dis Child Fetal Neonatal Ed* 2014; **99**: F240–F244.

Case 41

Hilary Humphreys

Case history

A 25-year-old female, who is 36 weeks pregnant, presents to a local maternity unit. Over the last 24 hours, she has developed fever, malaise, and some backache. She also has moderate to severe headache but does not have photophobia or vomiting. She underwent an appendectomy at 15 years of age and has otherwise been well. On examination, she has a tachycardia of 120/min, a temperature of 39.5 °C but there are no signs of meningism or other abnormal findings. She has a white cell count of 16,000/µl (4–11) with neutrophilia (80%) and a CRP of 120 (< 10 mg/L). She is admitted and blood cultures from her grow Gram-positive bacilli suggestive of *Listeria monocytogenes*. She is initially treated empirically for sepsis which is subsequently modified according to the results of culture and antibiotic susceptibility studies on the *L. monocytogenes*.

Questions

41.1 Outline some key biological and other features of *Listeria* spp. that may contribute to infection and assist in its identification in the laboratory.

41.2 What physiological and immunological changes during pregnancy may facilitate infection due to listeria?

41.3 What factors are associated with an increased risk of listeriosis?

41.4 What is the definitive treatment for invasive listeriosis during pregnancy?

41.5 What approaches are taken to preventing listeriosis during pregnancy?

Answers

41.1 Outline some key biological and other features of *Listeria* spp. that may contribute to infection and assist in its identification in the laboratory.

L. monocytogenes is a small Gram-positive facultative anaerobic rod or bacillus. It produces β-haemolysis on blood agar, which is due to the presence of a potential virulence factor listeriolysin, but its presence does not correlate with the severity of infection. This bacterium colonizes approximately 5% of healthy individuals usually in the gastrointestinal tract, but its isolation from sterile sites such as blood and cerebrospinal fluid (CSF) is always significant. The ability of the bacterium to grow at 4 °C and in high salt concentrations is used in the laboratory to aid in isolation and may partly explain its persistence in foodstuffs, in the environment, and in the gastrointestinal tract of humans and animals.

41.2 What physiological and immunological changes during pregnancy may facilitate infection due to listeria?

There are significant changes in sex hormones, T-cells, and cytokine activity during a normal healthy pregnancy. Levels of progesterone increase during pregnancy with the highest levels occurring during the third trimester. Progesterone alters the balance between T-helper 1 and T-helper 2 responses. Phagocytic activity increases during pregnancy as do the levels of several cytokines including interleukin-10 and granulocyte colony-stimulating factor. Conversely, both CD4 and CD8 cells decrease during pregnancy.

Listeria has a predilection for the placenta and foetus, and invasive listeriosis is much more frequent during pregnancy than in the general population. The placenta is a protective environment for bacterial growth with the formation of microabscesses from which listeria may spread to the bloodstream. Cell-to-cell spread of listeria also occurs and is largely independent of antibodies, complement, and neutrophils. Listeria activates T-cell-mediated immunity which through cytokines, attracts macrophages, resulting in granulomata formation where the bacteria are destroyed. Alterations in memory T-cells, which normally provide acquired resistance to listeriosis, may explain why this bacterium has a predisposition to causing infection in at-risk patients.

41.3 What factors are associated with an increased risk of listeriosis?

In addition to pregnancy, there is an increased risk of listeriosis in patients with:

+ leukaemia
+ other malignancies

- solid organ transplantation
- acquired immunodeficiency syndrome (AIDS)
- chronic conditions such as end-stage renal disease
- alcoholism
- diabetes mellitus
- patients on immunosuppressive therapy such as corticosteroids

It is mainly a food-borne infection and most cases are sporadically acquired in the community but nosocomial outbreaks have been described. Food associated with listeria includes soft cheeses, paté, smoked seafood, cantaloupe, and cold deli meats (Fig. 41.1). There may also be variations between ethnic groups and their risk of acquiring infection. For example, during pregnancy, listeriosis is more common amongst Hispanic women in the United States than in other ethnic groups. In the United Kingdom, the incidence has increased amongst ethnic groups in recent years and may be associated with the consumption of certain foods.

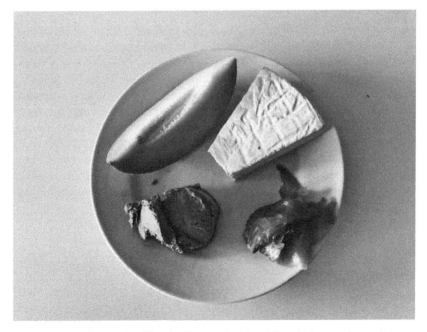

Figure 41.1 Well-recognized foodstuffs associated with listeriosis: cantaloupe, brie cheese, smoked salmon. and paté.

Reproduced courtesy of Niall Stevens, Department of Clinical Microbiology, RCSI, Ireland.

41.4 What is the definitive treatment for invasive listeriosis during pregnancy?

No randomized controlled trials have been undertaken in the management of listeria during pregnancy or in the treatment of bloodstream infection, meningitis, and endocarditis outside pregnancy. Most treatment recommendations are based upon *in-vitro* susceptibility testing or animal models. However, *L. monocytogenes* is resistant to cephalosporins and clindamycin with reduced susceptibility to chloramphenicol. It is susceptible to penicillins including ampicillin/amoxicillin which cross the placenta. In the laboratory, synergy has been demonstrated between ampicillin/amoxicillin and aminoglycosides such as gentamicin. Consequently, these two antibiotics are often used in combination but it is unclear if the aminoglycoside is really necessary. Alternative agents, particularly in patients allergic to β-lactam antibiotics, include macrolides, and co-trimoxazole, which achieves good serum and CSF concentrations. Treatment for 14 days is generally recommended but once the patient clinically settles, intravenous antibiotics can be replaced with equivalent oral agents.

41.5 What approaches are taken to preventing listeriosis during pregnancy?

Education is key in terms of informing pregnant mothers of where listeria can be found and how to avoid acquisition. Preventative measures include good practice regarding the provision of safe food to prevent all causes of food-borne illnesses such as appropriate storage of food, separating uncooked from cooked foods in the refrigerator, washing hands and cooking implements after handling uncooked foods, and the avoidance of specific foods associated with listeria during pregnancy. These foods include cold deli meats, soft cheeses such as feta and brie, paté or meat spreads, and smoked seafood including salmon. However, listeriosis has been associated with a broad range of foodstuffs, especially if inadequately stored or cleaned such as cantaloupe. Furthermore, it is important for the pregnant mother to avoid potentially contaminated food preparation surfaces even if she is not consuming any of the 'at-risk' foods herself.

Further reading

Kourtis AP, Read JS, Jamieson DJ. Pregnancy and infection. *New Engl J Med* 2014; **370**: 2211–18.

Madjunkov M, Chaudhry S, Ito S. Listeriosis during pregnancy. *Arch Gynaecol Obs* 2017; **296**: 143–52.

McCollum JT, Cronquist AB, Silk BJ, Jackson KA, O'Connor KA, et al. Multistate outbreak of listeriosis associated with cantaloupe. *New Engl J Med* 2013; **369**: 944–53.

Mook P, Grant KA, Little CL, Kafatos G, Gillespie IA. Emergence of pregnancy-related listeriosis amongst ethnic minorities in England and Wales. *Euro Surveillance* 2010; **15**: pii–19610.

Section 8

Miscellaneous infections

Case 42

Bridget L. Atkins

Case history

A 47-year-old man with type 2 diabetes mellitus on metformin and gliclazide is admitted via the acute medical take with a 3-week history of foot pain after walking with a hole in his shoe. For the previous 5 days he had developed increasing pain and redness between the first and second toes. His past medical history includes diabetic retinopathy.

On examination he is afebrile. He has right foot ulceration as shown in Fig. 42.1. The foot is swollen with erythema over the dorsum spreading to proximal midfoot region. Point-of-care glucose is 13 mmol/L. Bloods show a C-reactive protein (CRP) of > 156 mg/L and a neutrophilia (19.3 × 10^9/L). Serum creatinine is 56 with an estimated glomerular filtration rate of 56 ml/min/1.73m^2. Blood cultures are taken. A wound swab taken 2 days previously by his General Practitioner (GP) grew *Pseudomonas aeruginosa*, *Streptococcus agalactiae*, and *Streptococcus equisimilis*.

Questions

42.1 How should he be further assessed clinically?

42.2 What features in a diabetic foot may suggest a limb-threatening infection? What additional feature may be of concern in this patient?

42.3 What are the likely infecting organisms?

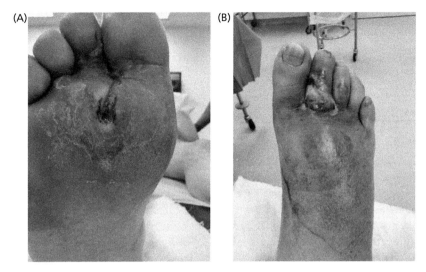

Figure 42.1 Photos of foot. (A) Plantar surface; (B) Dorsum of foot. (see colour plate)

Reproduced courtesy of Department of Microbiology and Infectious Diseases, John Radcliffe Hospital, Oxford, UK.

Answers

42.1 How should he be further assessed clinically?

He should be asked about any previous foot infections or ulcers, previous surgery to the foot, the quality of his personal diabetic foot care (use of footwear, recent trauma, daily inspections, podiatry review), and diabetic control. He should also be asked about the presence of neuropathy and any vascular assessments or reconstructions in the past. Examination should look for evidence of protective sensation (using a monofilament) and any other sensory loss or neuropathic deformity (Charcot arthropathy, claw or hammer toes, bunions, or callosities). Pulses should be examined, if necessary using on ward/clinic Doppler ultrasound. He should be examined generally for features of systemic sepsis and any other co-morbidities. He should have a plain radiograph looking for fractures, neuropathic changes, and any features suggesting osteomyelitis. An urgent magnetic resonance image (MRI) should be considered if it will affect surgical planning.

42.2 What features in a diabetic foot may suggest a limb-threatening infection? What additional feature may be of concern in this patient?

Box 42.1 describes clinical features that suggest a severe limb-threatening infection that needs urgent surgical assessment. This patient had none of these features at presentation.

In this patient there was an infected ulcer on the plantar surface with evidence of infection on the dorsum of the foot. This is a sign that there is likely to be deep infection with pus tracking upwards through the foot. Infection is likely to be significantly more extensive than is visualized externally.

42.3 What are the likely infecting organisms?

Many studies describing the microbiology of diabetic foot infections (DFIs) are flawed in that inappropriate specimens have been taken for culture. Superficial swabs may isolate multiple but colonizing organisms. Although obtaining swab specimens is convenient, results do not accurately represent deep infecting organisms, particularly if the wound has not been properly debrided. Tissue specimens obtained by biopsy, ulcer curettage, or aspiration are preferable to wound swab specimens.

S. aureus is the most common pathogen cultured from deep samples in most DFIs. Streptococci are also common especially in acute soft tissue infections. Gram-negative bacilli can be present—mostly commonly, *Escherichia coli, Klebsiella pneumoniae,* and *Proteus* spp., followed by *P. aeruginosa.* Obligate anaerobes (*Peptostreptococcus, Peptococcus,* and *Finegoldia magna*) may also be present.

Box 42.1 Signs of a possibly imminently limb-threatening infection

- ◆ Evidence of systemic inflammatory response
- ◆ Rapid progression of infection
- ◆ Extensive necrosis or gangrene
- ◆ Crepitus on examination or tissue gas on imaging
- ◆ Extensive ecchymoses or petechiae
- ◆ Extensive bony destruction, especially midfoot/hindfoot
- ◆ Failure of infection to improve with appropriate therapy
- ◆ Bullae, especially haemorrhagic
- ◆ New-onset wound anaesthesia
- ◆ Pain out of proportion to clinical findings
- ◆ Recent loss of neurologic function
- ◆ Critical limb ischaemia
- ◆ Extensive soft tissue loss

In clinical settings with less advanced healthcare available, lesser degrees of infection severity may make an infection limb-threatening.

Reproduced with permission from Lipsky BA, Berendt AR, Cornia PB, Pile JC, Peters EJ et al. Infectious Diseases Society of America clinical practice guideline for the diagnosis and treatment of diabetic foot infections. *Clin Infect Dis.* 2012 Jun;54(12):e132–73. DOI: 10.1093/cid/cis346.

Case history continued

He has palpable dorsalis pedis and posterior tibial pulses. He is assessed (using the Infectious Diseases Society of America (IDSA) classification) as having a severe infection (with low risk of methicillin-resistant *Staphylococcus aureus* (MRSA)) so he is commenced on intravenous piperacillin-tazobactam.

Over the next 48 hours the infection in his foot fails to settle and observations demonstrate fevers unresponsive to antibiotics. Soft tissue necrosis develops in the second toe and the erythema/cellulitis does not recede. Plain radiographs show no bony destruction but a small amount of gas in the soft tissues. MRI shows osteomyelitis but extensive soft tissue oedema and considerable fluid around the peroneus brevis tendon just proximal to its attachment.

Question

42.4 What is important next in the management of this patient?

Answer

42.4 What is important next in the management of this patient?

The clinical features now indicate a limb-threatening infection. He requires urgent debridement surgery by a surgeon skilled in managing DFIs.

Case history continued

He goes to theatre and considerable pus and necrotic soft tissue spreading to the metatarsal phalangeal joints are found. There are abscesses on the plantar side and dorsum of the foot the latter extending around the second and third extensor tendons. Debridement continues until it becomes apparent that he needs a trans-metatarsal amputation. It is felt he may need a subsequent below-knee amputation; however, with a repeat debridement 72 hours later the rest of the foot is ultimately saved. All samples grow *Streptococcus dysgalactiae*.

Question

42.5   How should he be managed in the longer term?

Answer

42.5 How should he be managed in the longer term?

Patients with diabetic foot ulcers (with or without infection) need a multidisciplinary team approach involving podiatrists, orthotists, endocrinologists, vascular surgeons, foot and ankle surgeons, and infection specialists. They require mechanical off-loading of established ulcerated areas and areas prone to ulceration in deformed (neuropathic) feet and appropriate footwear and/or orthoses. They need good diabetic control, a vascular assessment, and discussion of re-vascularization options if appropriate. When definite infection is present, appropriate clinical assessment and diagnostic investigations are essential. Antibiotics need to be used rationally and as specifically as possible. Over-use in uninfected ulcers is common. Semi-elective surgery may be required for underlying osteomyelitis and, in the longer term, elective surgery may be indicated for deformity. Patients need education and support for daily foot care and diabetic control.

Further reading

International Best Practice Guidelines : Wound management in diabetic foot ulcers. *Wounds International* 2013. Available at: https://www. woundsinternational.com.

Lipsky BA, Berendt AR, Cornia PB, Pile JC, Peters EJ, et al. Infectious Diseases Society of America. 2012 Infectious Diseases Society of America clinical practice guideline for the diagnosis and treatment of diabetic foot infections. *Clin Infect Dis* 2012; **54**: e132–e173.

Malhotra R, Chan CS, Nather A. Osteomyelitis in the diabetic foot. *Diabet Foot Ankle* 2014; **5**. https://www.ncbi.nlm.nih.gov/pmc/articles/PMC4119293/pdf/DFA-5-24445.pdf.

van Asten SA, La Fontaine J, Peters EJ, Bhavan K, Kim PJ, et al. The microbiome of diabetic foot osteomyelitis. *Eur J Clin Microbiol Infect Dis* 2016; **35**: 293–8.

Schaper NC, Van Netten JJ, Apelqvist J, Lipsky BA, Bakker K; International Working Group on the Diabetic Foot (IWGDF). Prevention and management of foot problems in diabetes: A Summary Guidance for Daily Practice 2015, based on the IWGDF guidance documents. *Diabetes Res Clin Pract* 2017;**124**: 84–92. doi: 10.1016/j.diabres.2016.12.007. Epub 2016 Dec 18.

Case 43

Lucinda Barrett and Bridget L. Atkins

Case history

A 44-year-old man presents to the Emergency Department (ED) with 2 days of fever and a painful right knee. On examination he is febrile 38.9 °C, tachycardic, and hypotensive with a swollen, warm right knee joint. Three years previously he had undergone a right total knee arthroplasty for post-traumatic arthritis. Two weeks previously he visited his General Practitioner (GP) with mild pain and swelling in the knee after a minor fall. A plain radiograph at that time showed a joint effusion but no bony or prosthesis abnormalities. There is no other past medical history.

Questions

43.1 What is the likely diagnosis and how can the presentation of this condition be classified?

43.2 What investigations should be performed?

43.3 What is the case definition for this condition?

43.4 What are the principles of the management of this condition?

Answers

43.1 What is the likely diagnosis and how can the presentation of this condition be classified?

This patient has a prosthetic joint infection (PPJI) of the right knee with features of systemic sepsis. PPJI is classified as 'early' when presentation is within 3 months of implantation, 'delayed' when presenting between 3 and 24 months, and 'late' if presenting beyond 2 years. Presentation may also be 'acute' (as in this patient) or 'chronic'. In chronic PPJI, patients complain of pain (if the prosthesis is loose this is often 'start-up' pain), a sinus tract may develop, and X-rays may show loosening of the prosthesis. Chronic infection is demonstrably present in around 15% of joint revisions for loosening.

43.2 What investigations should be performed?

In addition to blood cultures, a full blood count (FBC), renal and liver function, and inflammatory markers (CRP) should be taken. A plain radiograph of his knee should be performed to exclude a fracture and to look for loosening or displacement of the prosthesis. If there is doubt about the diagnosis of PPJI, an ultrasound can be performed to look for joint effusion and to aspirate fluid for microbiological culture. Synovial fluid Gram stain has low sensitivity for PPJI. Synovial fluid biomarkers such as leucocyte esterase, α-defensin, or CRP are controversial but may help with the diagnosis of PPJI when it is not certain. In more chronic cases a synovial fluid leucocyte count may be helpful. In culture-negative cases, molecular diagnostics such as 16s PCR may be considered. Research is ongoing as to the role of method such as metagenomic sequencing.

Given there are obvious clinical features of sepsis and joint infection, he needs urgent referral to orthopaedics for surgical intervention. In surgery, several intraoperative samples from different sites, each taken with separate sterile surgical instruments, should be sent for microbiological and histological analysis. Microbiological standard operating procedures need to include a method for disrupting biofilm and for resuscitating organisms (enrichment broths or blood culture bottles with prolonged cultures).

43.3 What is the case definition for this condition?

Many studies prior to 2011 lacked a gold standard definition for prosthetic joint infection. The Musculoskeletal Infection Society (MSIS) in the United States published a definition for PPJI in 2011 which was updated in 2018 (see Table 43.1). The definition has also been debated and modified at 2 International Consensus Meetings (ICM). Further refinement is likely from international authorities in the near future. In common they pre-operative criteria such as a discharging sinus, cultures positive joint aspirates, synovial fluid and serum biomarkers as well as results from intra-operative cultures and histology.

Table 43.1 The 2018 Musculoskeletal Infection Society (MSIS) definition of PPJI

Major criteria (at least one of the following)	Decision
Two positive cultures of the same organism	Infected
Sinus tract with evidence of communication to the joint or visualization of the prosthesis	

		Minor Criteria	Score	Decision
Preoperative Diagnosis	Serum	Elevated CRP *or* D-Dimer	2	>6 Infected **2–5 Possibly Infected**[a] 0–1 Not Infected
		Elevated ESR	1	
	Synovial	Elevated synovial *WBC count or LE*	3	
		Positive alpha-defensin	3	
		Elevated synovial PMN (%)	2	
		Elevated synovial CRP	1	

		Inconclusive pre-op score *or* dry tap[a]	Score	Decision
Intraoperative Diagnosis		Preoperative score	–	>6 Infected **4–5 Inconclusive**[b] <3 Not Infected
		Positive histology	3	
		Positive purulence	3	
		Single positive culture	2	

Reproduced with permission from Parvizi J. et al. (2018). The 2018 Definition of Periprosthetic Hip and Knee Infection: An Evidence-Based and Validated Criteria. *J Arthroplasty* 33(5):1309–1314.e2. DOI: 10.1016/j.arth.2018.02.078

43.4 What are the principles of the management of this condition?

The patient requires emergency surgery and broad-spectrum antibiotics. The first priority in this septic patient is to drain pus. In the case of acutely septic patients, an emergency arthroscopic or open wash-out may be required as an interim measure until a more definitive procedure can be undertaken. The IDSA 2012 guidelines recommend that if a patient presents within 1 month of implantation, or later following implantation but with < 3 weeks of symptoms, has a well-fixed prosthesis, and no evidence of a sinus tract, debridement, antibiotics, and implant retention (DAIR) should be considered. Many authorities consider DAIRs as an option for any well-fixed prosthesis provided soft tissue closure (primary or with a muscle flap) can be achieved at the end of surgery. The case discussed here meets these criteria. Modular components should be exchanged during a DAIR procedure. With appropriate antimicrobial therapy, success rates for DAIR (knee and hip arthroplasty) of around

75–80% (free of infection recurrence at 3 years) are reported. A DAIR should be performed by a senior orthopaedic surgeon skilled in the procedure.

The other surgical strategies in PPJI (especially chronic cases with failing implants) are revision of the prosthesis in one or two stages, removal of the prosthesis without re-implantation (hips), joint fusion (knees), or, in some cases with multiple relapses, poor soft tissues, and/or multi-drug resistant organisms, amputation. A two-stage revision is where the infected prosthesis is removed and usually a spacer is inserted to maintain limb anatomy. A new prosthesis is then inserted at a second operation, typically after several weeks of antibiotic therapy. A one-stage revision should be regarded as two stages under one anaesthetic. Stage 1 involves opening the joint, taking samples, removing the prosthesis and debriding all infected or abnormal tissue. Stage 2 includes new gloves and gowns, re-draping, and then re-implantation. The timing of antibiotics in a one-stage revision is controversial—antibiotics can be given after sampling to optimize the microbiological diagnosis rather than beforehand to maximize the chances of positive culture. This still allows high levels of antibiotics at the surgical site prior to stage 2—implantation of the new prosthesis—when it is critical to have eradicated any infected material or tissue. Some advocate earlier administration as the effect of one dose of antibiotics on the sensitivity of microbiological sampling may be minimal.

A one-stage revision for chronic infection has lower morbidity, requires one anaesthetic, and has a similar success rate to two-stage revisions in observational studies. It is favoured by several experts; however, a two-stage revision should still be considered in some patients such as those with antimicrobial resistant organisms, fungal infections, and/or immunosuppressed.

Patient co-morbidities, operative risk, and preference should also be taken into account. Some patients with chronic infections would prefer to live with a discharging sinus than risk further surgery that may reduce mobility. Long-term antibiotics alone may have a role in a minority of patients.

In the context of previously failed procedures, severe deformity, or where there is little chance of functional gain, amputation may be the best option.

In all cases the patient should be appropriately assessed and counselled by an orthopaedic surgeon experienced in managing infections, taking into account the patient's wishes, aims and expectations.

Case history continued

This patient has an acute infection and undergoes an urgent open joint debridement, including exchange of the rotating hinge liner (DAIR). Blood cultures taken in the ED are positive for methicillin-susceptible *Staphylococcus aureus* (MSSA). Intra-operative samples also grew MSSA with a similar antibiotic susceptibility profile, resistant to amoxicillin only.

Questions

43.5 Is *Staphylococcus aureus* a typical pathogen in this scenario? What other organisms commonly cause prosthetic joint infections?

43.6 What other investigations should be considered?

43.7 What post operative antimicrobial therapy should this patient receive?

43.8 For how long should he be treated?

Answers

43.5 Is *Staphylococcus aureus* a typical pathogen in this scenario? What other organisms commonly cause prosthetic joint infections?

Yes. Staphylococci are the causative organisms in around 50% of PPJI, with roughly equal proportions due to *S. aureus* and coagulase-negative species such as *S. epidermidis*. Streptococci, enterococci, and diphtheroids are isolated in 5–10% cases each while Gram negatives collectively account for around 10%. Polymicrobial cultures are seen in 15% while no pathogen is found in a minority. Fungal and mycobacteria are rare causes.

Inoculation of skin flora at the time of implantation is thought to underlie 'early/delayed' presentation, but with a 'late acute' presentation, the pathogenesis is typically due to haematogenous seeding in the context of bloodstream infection, with *S. aureus* being the most commonly isolated organism. Acute joint inflammation reflects the presence of numerous free-living (planktonic) bacteria, whereas more indolent symptoms are produced by the chronic presence of a lower number of sessile (adherent) organisms which are in slow growth phase. They are able to evade host defences by the ability to persist intracellularly and/or the excretion of extracellular polymeric substances (EPS) forming a biofilm.

43.6 What other investigations should be considered?

In the context of a *Staphylococcus aureus* bloodstream infection, clinical examination should look for any other possible sites of infection. Even in the absence of a heart murmur, there is a possibility of infective endocarditis and at the least, a transthoracic echocardiogram should be performed.

43.7 What post operative antimicrobial therapy should this patient receive?

Broad spectrum antibiotics should be rationalized as soon as culture results are available. In this case, he should be treated with high doses of an intravenous anti-staphylococcal penicillin (e.g. flucloxacillin). Assuming susceptibility to rifampicin, and the absence of contraindications, this should be added when source control has been fully achieved and when drains have been removed (usually at a dose of 300–450 mg twice daily orally). Traditionally, intravenous therapy is continued for up to 6 weeks post-operatively, however many clinicians now favour changing to highly bioavailable oral agents at an early stage unless there is a *S. aureus* bloodstream infection. The OVIVA trial demonstrated non-inferiority of early oral antibiotics in bone and joint infections (but excluded *S. aureus* bloodstream infection). In staphylococcal PPJIs, a rifampicin-containing regimen is preferred when possible, for example with a fluoroquinolone, doxycycline, fusidic acid, or co-trimoxazole. It is important to review all other medications as significant interactions with, for example, anticoagulants, antidepressants, antiepileptic agents are common.

In staphylococcal PPJIs, a rifampicin-containing regimen is preferred when possible, for example with a fluoroquinolone, doxycycline, fusidic acid, or co-trimoxazole. It is important to review all other medications as significant interactions with, for example, anticoagulants, antidepressants, antiepileptic agents are common.

43.8 For how long should he be treated?

The duration of antibiotics after a DAIR is controversial. Many recommend oral therapy for 3–6 months from the date of surgery but robust clinical trials are required. Frequent monitoring of FBC, renal and liver function, and CRP is required during antibiotic therapy, alongside clinic follow-up to ensure clinical progression and the absence of significant side effects.

Clinical trials are also required to determine the duration of antibiotics after the first stage of a two-stage revision (most give 6 weeks and then have an antibiotic free interval prior to re-implantation) and a one-stage revision (most give 3 months). An early switch to bioavailable, well tolerated, oral antibiotics should be considered in many patients.

Further reading

Li HK, Rombach I, Zambellas R, Walker AS, McNally MA, et al. OVIVA Trial Collaborators. Oral versus intravenous antibiotics for bone and joint infection. *N Engl J Med* 2019; **380**: 425–36.

Osmon DR, Berbari EF, Berendt AR, Lew D, Zimmerli W, et al. Diagnosis and management of prosthetic joint infection: clinical practice guidelines by the Infectious Diseases Society of America. *Clin Infect Dis* 2013; **56**: 1–25.

Public Health England, Standards for microbiology investigations (SMI) Investigation of orthopaedic implant associated infections. Available at: https://www.gov.uk/government/publications/smi-b-44-investigation-of-prosthetic-joint-infection-samples.

Senneville E, Joulie D, Legout L, Valette M, Dezèque H, et al. Outcome and predictors of treatment failure in total hip/knee prosthetic joint infections due to *Staphylococcus aureus*. *Clin Infect Dis* 2011; **53**: 334–40.

Zimmerli W, Frei R, Widmer AF, Rajacic Z. Microbiological tests to predict treatment outcome in experimental device-related infections due to *Staphylococcus aureus*. *J Antimicrob Chemother* 1994; **33**: 959–67.

Case 44

William L. Irving

Case history

A doctor is asked to attend the hospital's Occupational Health (OH) department on the first day of her new appointment on a training programme in orthopaedic surgery in the UK. She is UK-born and trained at a London teaching hospital.

Questions

44.1 What is an exposure-prone procedure (EPP)?

44.2 What tests would the OH department initiate to satisfy themselves that the trainee is fit to practise EPPs within the NHS Trust (hospital)?

44.3 What precautions would the OH department take when organizing these tests?

Answers

44.1 What is an exposure-prone procedure (EPP)?

An exposure-prone procedure (EPP) is defined as an invasive procedure where there is a risk that injury to the healthcare worker may result in the exposure of the patient's open tissues to the healthcare worker's blood—and therefore there is a risk of healthcare worker-to-patient transmission of a blood-borne virus. Such procedures are common in orthopaedic surgery.

44.2 What tests would the OH department initiate to satisfy themselves that the trainee is fit to practise EPPs within the NHS Trust (hospital)?

Healthcare workers infected with a blood-borne virus may transmit their infection to patients. For the protection of patients, healthcare workers coming in to the National Health Service (NHS) who wish to perform EPPs have to agree to being tested for evidence of infection with hepatitis B virus (HBV), hepatitis C virus (HCV), and human immunodeficiency virus (HIV).

44.3 What precautions would the OH department take when organizing these tests?

The OH department would need to send an identified validated sample (IVS) to the laboratory for testing. This involves the healthcare worker providing photographic proof of identity, the sample being taken in the OH department, and then delivered to the laboratory by the usual manner (i.e. not transported by the healthcare worker). These somewhat draconian instructions are necessary as infected healthcare workers have 'faked' negative results by substituting someone else's sample for their own on more than one occasion, an offence which has subsequently resulted in them being struck off by the UK General Medical Council and receiving a gaol sentence.

Case history continued

Further discussions reveal that she will be undertaking EPPs. She is counselled about what might occur depending on various results, and especially if these are positive. She is particularly keen to complete her training in orthopaedic surgery and to sub-specialize in knee surgery including knee reconstructive surgery.

Question

44.4 Under what circumstances (if any) could this trainee be allowed to undertake EPPs if she was

a.   Hepatitis B surface-antigen positive?

b.   Anti-HCV positive?

c.   Anti-HIV positive?

Answer

44.4 Under what circumstances (if any) could this trainee be allowed to undertake EPPs if she was

a. Hepatitis B surface-antigen positive?

b. Anti-HCV positive?

c. Anti-HIV positive?

a. The presence of hepatitis B surface antigen means that the source individual is infected with hepatitis B virus. The laboratory would proceed to define the nature of the infection in greater detail. If this is a chronic infection (most likely, and defined by being IgM (immunoglobulin M) anti-HBc negative), then the HBe antigen/anti-HBe status and the viral load (in IU/ml) in peripheral blood would be determined. Guidance up until July 2019 decreed that HBe antigen positive healthcare workers were not allowed to perform EPPs under any circumstances. Anti-HBe positive healthcare workers were allowed to perform EPPs provided that their viral load was below 200 IU/ml, either through natural suppression, or as the result of taking antiviral therapy, in the latter case provided that their pre-treatment viral load did not exceed 20,000 IU/ml. However, with the advent of more potent anti-HBV drugs with high barriers to resistance (tenofovir and entecavir), new regulations issued in July 2019 allow any HBV-infected healthcare worker to perform EPPs irrespective of their HBeAg/anti-HBe status, provided that their viral load is less than 200 IU/ml. For those who achieve this through natural suppression, monitoring of viral load is every 12 months. Those who achieve this through anti-viral therapy must be monitored every 12 weeks. The responsibility for such monitoring lies with the occupational health department.

b. Anti-HCV positivity means that the source individual has been infected with HCV. Any such sample should automatically be tested for HCV RNA to determine whether or not the infection has been cleared. Individuals who are anti-HCV positive, HCV RNA negative are not infectious—the best evidence for this comes from blood transfusion lookbacks, where donations from such individuals have been shown not to transmit infection. Thus, there are no restrictions on EPPs for any healthcare worker with this profile. Hence this doctor could complete her training in orthopaedic surgery. However, the presence of HCV RNA in a peripheral blood sample indicates current infection and there are many reports of healthcare workers-to-patient transmission of HCV arising from HCV RNA-positive healthcare workers. Whilst it is likely that the infectivity of such an individual will be dependent on viral load, in contrast to the situation with HBV, there are no data on the viral loads in healthcare workers responsible for transmission, and therefore no evidence base upon which to set a viral load cut-off below which healthcare workers can be allowed to proceed with EPPs. Thus, if the trainee were found to be anti-HCV positive, HCV RNA positive, she would not be allowed to carry out EPPs. The good news is that with the new, direct-acting antiviral agents (DAAs), it is highly likely

(> 95%) that her infection could be cured (again, in stark contrast to HBV), and she would be allowed to perform EPPs if she was shown to be HCV RNA negative 24 weeks after the end of her treatment course (8 or 12 weeks depending upon HCV genotype and underlying liver disease status).

    c. Anti-HIV positivity means that the healthcare worker is infected with HIV, and therefore the possibility of healthcare worker-to-patient transmission must be considered. In the world literature to date, there are four healthcare workers associated with such transmissions—from an orthopaedic surgeon to one patient, a gynaecologist to one patient, a nurse to one patient with an unclear history of EPPs having been performed, and the Florida dentist who transmitted HIV to 6 patients, although the precise circumstances of that last event have never been clarified. Whilst there was an initial reluctance to allow HIV-infected healthcare workers to perform EPPs for a number of reasons, the paucity of recorded transmissions, and accumulated evidence from a large number of lookback exercises (where patients treated by a healthcare worker subsequently shown to be HIV-infected have been recalled for testing) involving tens of thousands of patients, revealing no further transmissions, has led to a more evidence-based approach. Guidelines introduced in the United Kingdom in 2014 now allow HIV-infected healthcare workers to perform EPPs as long as (i) they are on combination anti-retroviral therapy and have a plasma viral load suppressed to < 200 copies/ml; (ii) are under the joint supervision of an OH consultant as well as their treating physician; and (iii) their viral load is monitored strictly every 3 months.

Further reading

Incident Investigation Team and others. Transmission of hepatitis B to patients from four infected surgeons without hepatitis B e antigen. *New Eng J Med* 1997; **336**: 178–84.

Public Health England. Integrated guidance on health clearance of healthcare workers and the management of healthcare workers infected with bloodborne viruses (hepatitis B, hepatitis C and HIV) October 2017 Available at: https://www.gov.uk/government/publications/bbvs-in-healthcare-workers-health-clearance-and-management.

Rajoriya N, Combet C, Zoulim F, Janssen HLA. How viral genetic variants and genotypes influence disease and treatment outcome of chronic hepatitis B. Time for an individualised approach? *J Hepatol* 2017; **67**: 1281–97.

Case 45

Andrew Woodhouse

Case history

A 32-year-old nurse who has been working as a volunteer in a hospital in rural Nigeria for 6 months presents to the Emergency Department (ED) complaining of 3 days of fever (self-recorded up to 38.5 °C) and myalgia, headache, and fatigue. She arrived back in the United Kingdom a week prior to the development of fever. During the period she was working in Nigeria she was relatively well apart from occasional episodes of diarrhoea. She took malaria prophylaxis with doxycyline for the first 3 months of her trip but donated the remaining antibiotics to one of the outreach clinics attached to the hospital in which she worked. She was not aware of any patients that she cared for having confirmed viral haemorrhagic fever (VHF) and does not recall any needlestick injuries or episodes of inadvertent exposure to blood or body fluids. Examination confirms fever and tachycardia with normal blood pressure. No rash is evident. Exam is otherwise normal.

Questions

45.1 What illnesses need to be considered in the differential diagnosis in this case?

45.2 What advice should be given to the Emergency Department (ED)?

45.3 What diagnostics will help to establish or refute a diagnosis of VHF?

45.4 What precautions need to be taken in the use of personal protective equipment (PPE) in caring for patients with possible VHF?

45.5 What treatment is available for VHFs?

Answers

45.1 What illnesses need to be considered in the differential diagnosis in this case?

The differential diagnosis in this case is broad as her presenting features are relatively non-specific. The possibilities encompass a range of infections that could be acquired in rural Nigeria including malaria, enteric fever, rickettsial infection, and a number of viral infections including viral haemorrhagic fevers. Prior to the recent Ebola Virus Disease (EVD) outbreak in Sierra Leone, Guinea, and Liberia in the mid-2010s, the VHF most commonly considered in patients returning from West Africa, albeit very rarely, was Lassa fever. Lassa virus is a member of the Arenaviridae family. It is endemic in West Africa including Nigeria, where it was first described, although it is rare and the distribution of disease and occurrence of cases is not evenly spread throughout the country. Further information about her work location and whether any Lassa fever cases have been diagnosed in that area is important.

45.2 What advice should be given to the ED?

A careful risk assessment is essential when considering the possibility of VHF in a patient with fever returning from an endemic country. Hospitals should have an easily accessible policy and guidance for the assessment of possible VHF cases. This policy should link in and be consistent with national guidance. In the absence of an outbreak situation the likelihood of VHF is low and risk assessment helps to determine an appropriate management pathway. Risk factors to explore in Lassa fever include having spent time in rural settings and possible contact with infected rat urine or faeces, potentially via contaminated food. Another significant exposure risk is for healthcare workers who have been caring for patients with Lassa fever and had contact with contaminated body fluids or secretions. Given that Lassa fever can be asymptomatic or a relatively mild illness, exposure in the healthcare setting may not be readily apparent, particularly in environments where there is limited diagnostic capacity.

Patients who, based on initial risk assessment, require VHF to be excluded should be isolated and staff should wear appropriate PPE when delivering care to the patient. It is critical that other, more likely diagnoses are rigorously sought including, in particular, malaria. The laboratory needs to be notified that samples have come from a possible VHF case so they can take appropriate handling precautions but initial sample processing should take place locally.

45.3 What diagnostics will help to establish or refute a diagnosis of VHF?

The most helpful test in the acute setting is reverse transcriptase polymerase chain reaction (RT-PCR) on blood. Virus specific serology may also be helpful but IgM antibody is found later in the illness compared to when virus can be detected using RT-PCR. Blood should be sent urgently to an appropriately accredited laboratory with the necessary isolation and containment facilities—usually a Category 4 pathogen laboratory in most high income countries. A system should be in place for the transport of samples from local hospitals to the reference laboratory. Many reference laboratories will run a panel of tests depending on the geographic area of the potential acquisition and in addition to relevant VHF RT-PCR they may include malaria, leptospirosis and rickettsia PCR tests. Other laboratory findings in VHF are non-specific but may include deranged liver enzymes, leucopaenia, and thrombocytopaenia.

45.4 What precautions need to be taken in the use of PPE in caring for patients with possible VHF?

The Ebola outbreak highlighted the importance of adhering to strict protocols and training in the use of PPE. A number of the documented cases of nosocomial transmission in the Ebola outbreak were felt to be due to breakdowns in following protocol in the use of PPE, particularly in the removal of contaminated equipment (doffing). Inadvertent exposure and inoculation via the face and eyes seemed to be a particular issue. Use of a checklist and the assistance of an observer as a 'buddy' during the process of donning (putting on) or doffing (removing) PPE is helpful in avoiding inadvertent lapses in infection control by healthcare workers.

45.5 What treatment is available for VHFs?

The mainstay of treatment for VHFs is supportive. Ebola and Marburg viruses are highly pathogenic with a potentially rapid clinical course. Aggressive supportive care with particular attention to resuscitation, fluid and electrolyte management, and replacement of blood products plus correction of coagulopathy is likely to have improved outcomes in the recent Ebola epidemic. Other treatment approaches tried during the recent Ebola outbreak included immunotherapy with convalescent plasma. Some monoclonal antibodies and a variety of experimental antiviral agents have been used on a compassionate basis. These include Mab114, REGN-EB3, ZMapp, remdesivir, and favipiravir. Although both types of interventions were used in a small number of patients treated in high income countries, any evidence of benefit is anecdotal rather than highly evidence-based.

Of the VHFs, Lassa virus is an exception in that ribavirin has shown useful antiviral activity. It is most effective when given early in the course of infection (within 6 days of illness onset) hence the need for rapid diagnostic test results. There is no specific pharmacological treatment for Marburg virus or Crimean Congo hemorrhagic fever.

Further reading

Beeching NJ, Fenech M, Houlihan CF. Ebola virus disease. *Br Med J* 2014; **349**: g7348.

Damon IK, Rollin PE, Choi MJ, Arthur RR, Redfield RR. New tools in the Ebola arsenal. *New Eng J Med* 2018; **379**: 1981–3.

Leblebicioglu H, Ozaras R, Fletcher TE, Beeching NJ. Crimean-Congo haemorrhagic fever in travellers: A systematic review. *Travel Med Infect Dis* 2016; **14**: 73–80.

Public Health England. Viral haemorrhagic fever: ACDP algorithm and guidance on management of patients. 2016. Available at: https://www.gov.uk/government/publications/viral-haemorrhagic-fever-algorithm-and-guidance-on-management-of-patients.

Racsa LD, Kraft Cs, Olinger GG, Hensley LE. Viral hemorrhagic fever diagnostics. *Clin Inf Dis* 2016; **62**: 214–19.

Case 46

Andrew Woodhouse

Case history

A 45-year-old woman received a simultaneous pancreas kidney transplant for diabetes and end-stage renal failure 6 months earlier. During work-up for her transplant she was found to be seronegative for cytomegalovirus (CMV). The donor from whom she received her transplant was seropositive for CMV.

Questions

46.1 What would be the recommended management following transplantation with respect to the CMV status of donor and recipient?

46.2 Would the recommendation be different if the recipient had been found to be CMV seropositive in her pre-transplant work-up?

46.3 Would any form of CMV preventive strategy be required if both recipient and donor were CMV seronegative?

Answers

46.1 What would be the recommended management following transplantation with respect to the CMV status of donor and recipient?

The situation described—donor positive, recipient negative CMV status (D+/R–)—places the recipient at high risk of developing symptomatic CMV infection and disease. In receiving an organ from a CMV-positive donor she is effectively undergoing a primary CMV infection. With no pre-existing CMV immunity, coupled with the immunosuppression required to prevent rejection she is very likely to develop high levels of CMV viraemia and subsequent disease involving her graft or other organs. It is recommended that such patients receive prophylactic treatment with antiviral agents in the immediate post-transplant period. Ganciclovir prophylaxis was the approach initially shown to be most effective in this situation but it has now largely been replaced by valganciclovir with its more favourable pharmacokinetics. Typically, a D+/R– patient would receive 900 mg of valganciclovir once daily orally for 3–6 months following transplantation. Longer prophylaxis durations have been recommended for certain situations with up to 12 months recommended by some guidelines for transplants with high levels of immunosuppression and high risk of CMV disease such as lung, multi-visceral, and small intestinal.

46.2 Would the recommendation be different if the recipient had been found to be CMV seropositive in her pre-transplant work-up?

Recipients with antibodies to CMV have had previous infection with the virus and hence have an existing humoral and cell-mediated immune response to CMV. A positive recipient of an organ from a positive donor (D+/R+) is still at risk of developing symptomatic CMV infection or disease but the risk is reduced compared to the D+/R– situation. Nonetheless, immunosuppression will abrogate the host immune response and in addition the pre-existing host immune response may be less effective at controlling donor CMV. In light of this, prophylaxis is still recommended by most guidelines in this situation with valganciclovir being favoured. A shorter duration of 3 months is usually recommended. If the donor were CMV-negative and the recipient positive (D–/R+) the risk of CMV infection or disease developing is lower. There is debate about the best approach in this situation. There is an argument that rather than universal prophylaxis, a monitoring and pre-emptive treatment strategy can be adopted. Regular blood testing for CMV, by antigen detection, or PCR is undertaken to monitor for evidence of early CMV reactivation. Once a specific viral load threshold is detected or a rapid rise in viral load is seen, pre-emptive treatment can be started, aiming to prevent the development of symptomatic infection or disease.

46.3 Would any form of CMV preventive strategy be required if both recipient and donor were CMV seronegative?

No pharmacological preventive strategy is required in this situation as neither graft nor host harbor latent CMV infection. Use of CMV-negative and leucocyte-depleted blood products in these patients is a primary preventive strategy.

Case history continued

The patient completes a 6-month course of prophylactic valganciclovir. Her post-transplant course has been uneventful and both grafts are functioning well. At the time of her transplant she received alemtuzumab (anti-CD52) as part of her induction immunosuppression and has had relatively little corticosteroid post transplant. Her current immunosuppression is mycophenolate and tacrolimus.

Eight months after transplant she presents to clinic complaining of abdominal pain, fevers, and intermittent diarrhoea for 2–3 weeks. Her graft function remains stable. No CMV viral load monitoring has been undertaken since completing valganciclovir. A CMV viral load is taken and shows a low level CMV viral load of 800 IU/ml plasma. Her full blood count (FBC) is normal. Faeces microscopy and culture does not demonstrate any bacterial or parasitic pathogen.

Questions

46.4 Is she still at risk of complications of CMV infection?

46.5 What could be done to reduce the risk of CMV complications during this later post-transplant period?

46.6 Is CMV a possible explanation for her current symptoms?

46.7 How can gastrointestinal CMV be proven or excluded?

Answers

46.4 Is she still at risk of complications of CMV infection?

Yes. There remains a risk of developing symptomatic CMV infection with potential organ involvement. The risk of developing what is termed 'late' CMV disease after completing a period of prophylaxis is difficult to quantify. It is likely to depend on a number of factors including the degree of CMV immunity a patient has developed while on valganciclovir suppression which will influence the ongoing net state of immunosuppression. Late CMV disease, occurring after the period of prophylaxis, can present either as a CMV syndrome with fever, viraemia, and cytopaenia or as end-organ disease.

Recipients of T-cell depleting antibodies are at increased risk of CMV reactivation. In the case of alemtuzumab, the increased risk is when it is used to treat rejection rather than its use in induction immunosuppression.

46.5 What could be done to reduce the risk of CMV complications during this later post-transplant period?

A monitoring approach can be adopted for high-risk patients who have completed a period of valganciclovir prophylaxis post transplant. Regular CMV viral load monitoring, typically once weekly, is undertaken with the opportunity to commence antiviral treatment if a significant viral load level is detected. The threshold for initiating treatment may vary between centres depending in part on the test used.

46.6 Is CMV a possible explanation for her current symptoms?

Yes. The viral load detected is low level but does indicate detectable virus in plasma. In the absence of recent prior viral loads it is not possible to know whether this is a recent development. A viral load of this magnitude is often asymptomatic and further regular CMV monitoring would be undertaken to help make decisions regarding treatment. Her abdominal symptoms raise the possibility of CMV disease involving the gastrointestinal tract. CMV enteritis and colitis can develop without a high plasma CMV viral load being detected.

46.7 How can gastrointestinal CMV be proven or excluded?

Colonoscopy can be undertaken which allows direct visualization and biopsy of the colon. Her symptoms suggest involvement of the lower gastrointestinal tract but CMV can involve any level. Esophagogastroduodenoscopy is also potentially useful and may demonstrate areas of focal ulceration and allows biopsies to be obtained. Biopsy material is sent for histopathology, including immunofluorescence staining. CMV PCR can also be undertaken on fresh tissue.

Case history continued

A colonoscopy is performed which demonstrates features of CMV colitis. (Fig. 46.1) A biopsy of the involved tissue shows CMV infection with evidence of viral inclusion bodies (Fig. 46.2).

Question

46.8 If CMV infection is confirmed, what treatment should be initiated and how long should treatment continue?

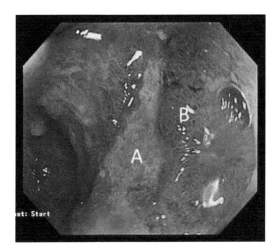

Figure 46.1 Colonoscopy showing features of CMV colitis. A mucosal ulcer (A) is surrounded by erythema (B) (see colour plate).

Reproduced courtesy of University Hospitals Birmingham NHS Foundation Trust, UK.

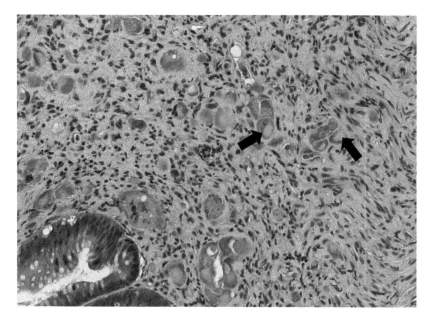

Figure 46.2 Cytomegalovirus colitis with multiple large infected endothelial and stromal cells in the lamina propria showing typical intranuclear inclusions (arrows). (H&E; ×200) (see colour plate).

Reproduced courtesy of University Hospitals Birmingham NHS Foundation Trust, UK.

Answer

46.8 If CMV infection is confirmed, what treatment should be initiated and how long should treatment continue?

Treatment with ganciclovir or valganciclovir should be started. Intravenous ganciclovir with a switch to oral valganciclovir when a treatment response is seen is a typical approach. Oral valganciclovir does have favourable pharmacokinetics though and has been shown to be as effective in the treatment of CMV disease in the solid organ transplant group.

If there are any concerns about absorption or in patients with severe disease or high viral loads then intravenous ganciclovir should be used initially. Treatment should continue until there is a clear clinical and virological response but needs to be individualized for each patient. A duration of at least 2–3 weeks is recommended by most authorities even in patients with a rapid response. Undetectable circulating virus at completion of therapy is associated with lower rates of relapse.

Further reading

Andrews PA, Emery VC, Newstead C. Summary of the British Transplantation Society Guidelines for the prevention and management of CMV disease after solid organ transplantation. *Transplant* 2011; **92**: 1181–7.

Kotton CN, Kumar D, Caliendo AM, Huprikar S, Chou S, et al. On behalf of The Transplantation Society International CMV Consensus Group. *Transplant* 2018; **102**: 900–31.

Lumbreras C, Manuel O, Len O, ten Berge IJ, Sgarabotto D, et al., on behalf of the ESCMID study group of infection in compromised hospitals (ESGICH). Cytomegalovirus infection in solid organ transplant recipients. *Clin Microbiol Infect* 2014; **20**: 19–26.

Marcelin JR, Beam E, Razunable RR. Cytomegalovirus in liver transplant recipients: Updates on clinical management. *World J Gastroenterol* 2014; **20**: 10658–67.

Razonable RR, Humar A, and the AST Infectious Diseases Community of Practice. Cytomegalovirus in solid organ transplantation. *Am J Transplant* 2013; **13**: 93–106.

Case 47

Hilary Humphreys

Case history

A 35-year-old female is admitted with a Glasgow Coma Scale (GCS) of 7 against a background of poorly controlled insulin-dependent diabetes mellitus. Initial investigations confirm diabetic ketoacidosis, thought to be precipitated by an infection. Following resuscitation and the administration of broad-spectrum anti-bacterial agents and caspofungin, she remains stable with a GCS of 15, but she continues to be pyrexial. A collateral history indicates that she has had symptoms consistent with sinusitis for a number of weeks before hospital admission, including nasal discharge, but more recently she is also having facial pain. On examination, she has peri-orbital cellulitis.

Questions

47.1 Given the background history and presentation, what opportunist infection may this may be?

47.2 What are the recognized risk factors for this condition?

47.3 How may this condition manifest?

Answers

47.1 Given the background history and presentation, what opportunist Infection may this may be?

Mucormycosis. This represents a spectrum of sub-acute, acute and often rapidly progressing infections, caused by angiotropic fungi of the order of Mucorales, and which are associated with a high mortality. While the sinusitis could be due to more common causes such as respiratory bacteria (e.g. non-capsulated *Haemophilus influenzae*), a background of poorly controlled diabetes mellitus and symptoms of sinusitis for some weeks with peri-orbital cellulitis should raise the possibility of this being mucormycosis, which in the setting here may be rapidly progressive.

47.2 What are the recognized risk factors for this condition?

This condition is associated with a range of malignant and other conditions although overall it is relatively uncommon even in these categories of patients (Table 47.1). Mucormycosis may also mimic aspergillosis, clinically and radiologically in the severely neutropenic patient, especially if presenting with respiratory symptoms and signs.

47.3 How may this condition manifest?

Pulmonary mucormycosis occurs most frequently in neutropenic patients. Rhinocerebral mucormycosis is the most common form found in patients with

Table 47.1 Risk factors for mucormycosis

Predisposing condition	Details
Malignancy	Acute myeloid leukaemia, post-stem cell transplantation Risk ~1%
Solid organ transplants	Renal, risk 0.2–1.2%, also liver and lung transplantation
Diabetes mellitus	Uncontrolled hyperglycaemia, ketoacidosis with poor social conditions
Iron overload	Iron chelation therapy, ketoacidosis (associated with increased free iron)
Others	Trauma—especially in warmer climates, e.g. India, and treatment may require amputation HIV/AIDS—intravenous drug use High-dose steroids—macrophage migration impaired Breakthrough infections in patients on antifungal prophylaxis (voriconazole and echinocandins)

diabetes mellitus. Persistent symptoms of sinusitis together with peri-orbital cellulitis, a black necrotic eschar on the palate, and cranial nerve palsies are very suggestive. Cutaneous mucormycosis arises from direct inoculation and is often localized especially if associated with trauma. Other forms of mucormycosis include gastrointestinal disease resulting in upper gastrointestinal bleeding or enterocolitis, disseminated infection, involving the brain and other organs, and finally localized infections of the endocardium and bone, although these are rare.

Case history continued

The patient does not respond to the broad-spectrum antibacterial agents and caspofungin. She undergoes MRI scanning, which shows significant abnormalities of the left maxillary sinus and orbit. This is followed by appropriate surgical intervention and antifungal treatment. She gradually improves but requires a long in-patient stay.

Questions

47.4 What are the main laboratory approaches to confirming the diagnosis of mucormycosis?

47.5 What are the treatment options for mucormycosis?

47.6 For how long should treatment be continued?

47.7 What is the overall mortality from this condition?

Answers

47.4 What are the main laboratory approaches to confirming the diagnosis of mucormycosis?

These include microscopy, culture, and molecular-based techniques. Serological methods are unreliable, especially in the immunocompromised, and fungal assays such as those for β D-glucan do not detect the main causes of mucormycosis which are *Rhizopus* spp., *Mucor* spp., and *Cunninghamella bertholletiae*. Direct microscopy or microscopy of tissue sections (Fig. 47.1) is required for definitive diagnosis. Tissue sections stained with Grocot, Gomori methenamine silver (GMS), or periodic acid-Schiff (PAS) stains may show large branching pauci-septate hyphae usually at a wide angle of 90°, but these may stain less deeply than for other invasive fungi such as aspergillosis. Matrix-assisted laser desorption ionization time-of-flight (MALDI-TOF) and molecular approaches, mainly based on PCR and often in-house assays or pan-fungal PCR assays, are increasingly being evaluated. However, these are often not available locally.

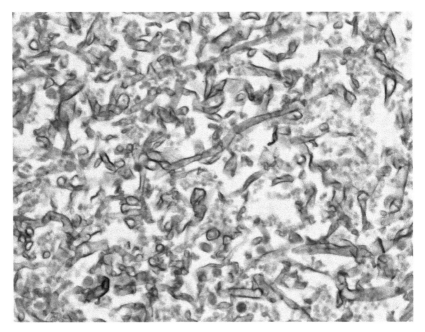

Figure 47.1 Fungal stain (Grocott) showing hyphae typical of mucormycosis (see colour plate).

Reproduced courtesy of Michael Farrell, Neuropathologist, Beaumont Hospital, Dublin, Ireland.

47.5 What are the treatment options for mucormycosis?

Extensive surgical debridement is usually necessary, including sometimes orbital exenteration. Debridement may need to be repeated on a number of occasions because of the destructive and necrotic nature of this condition hence hospital stay can be prolonged. Inadequate source control is often associated with a poor prognosis. On their own, echinocandins such as caspofungin, have no activity but they are sometimes used in combination. This may explain the failure of this patient to respond to caspofungin in addition to the need for surgery. The two most active agents *in vitro* are amphotericin B and posaconazole, the former usually administered in high dose. More recently, isavuconazole has recently been approved in the United States with some promising results. Adjunctive therapeutic approaches include hyperbarbic oxygen and iron chelating agents such as deferasirox (Table 47.2). Reducing the degree of immunosuppression, if possible, is also helpful such as by the administration of granulocyte (macrophage) colony-stimulating factors. However, as the condition is not common, randomized controlled trials are not available to provide definitive treatment guidelines. The available evidence is based on *in vitro* data and case series/reports.

47.6 For how long should treatment be continued?

Usually months of treatment are required but this will be governed by the underlying condition of the patient, the degree to which immunosuppression may be reversed, and the efficacy of the surgical approach. In most cases, however, a minimum of 6 months' treatment is probably required.

Table 47.2 Treatment options (excluding surgery) for mucormycosis

Agent/Approach	Comment
Amphothericin B	Lipid preparations to facilitate higher doses, e.g. up to 10 mg/kg/day and to minimize toxicity
Posaconazole	Not first-line therapy but good *in vitro* activity
Echinocandin	Only used in combination such as with amphotericin B
Isavuconazole	New azole agent with comparable *in vitro* activity to posaconazole
Hyperbaric oxygen	Adjunctive treatment: fungistatic but aids neovascularization
Deferasirox	Chelates iron; used with amphotericin B but efficacy is equivocal

47.7 What is the overall mortality from this condition?

A recent review of 851 individual cases found a mortality of 46% with the highest risk being in disseminated infection compared to cutaneous infection, which had the lowest risk for death. Also, the mortality from infection with *Cunninghamella* spp. was higher than from infections caused by other Mucorales.

Further reading

Jeong W, Keighley C, Wolfe R, Lee WL, Slavin MA, et al. The epidemiology and clinical manifestations of mucormycosis; a systematic review and meta-analysis of case reports. *Clin Microbiol Infect* 2019; **25**: 26–34.

Lackner M, Caramalho R, Lass-Flörl C. Laboratory diagnosis of mucromycosis: current status and future perspectives. *Fut Microbiol* 2014; **9**: 683–95.

Lelievre L, Garcia-Hermoso D, Abdoul H, Brignier AC, Sterkers M, et al. Posttraumatic murcormycosis. a nationwide study in France and review of the literature. *Medicine* 2014; **93**: 395–404.

Rapidis AD. Orbitomaxillary mucormycosis (zygomycosis) and the surgical approach to treatment: perspectives from a maxillofacial surgeon. *Clin Microbiol Infect* 2009; **15**: 98–102.

Spellberg B, Ibrahim A, Roilides E, Lewis RE, Lortholary O, et al. Combination therapy for mucromycosis: why, what and how? *Clin Infect Dis* 2012; **54**: S73–S78.

List of cases by diagnosis

Case 1 Cellulitis and other bacterial skin infections

Case 2 Toxic shock syndrome

Case 3 Chickenpox

Case 4 Measles

Case 5 Lyme disease

Case 6 Community-acquired pneumonia

Case 7 Acute exacerbation of chronic obstructive pulmonary disease (COPD)

Case 8 Influenza

Case 9 Severe imported respiratory infections

Case 10 Tuberculosis

Case 11 Whooping cough

Case 12 Lung infiltrate in the immunocompromised host

Case 13 Cystic fibrosis

Case 14 Cryptococcal infections

Case 15 Peritonitis

Case 16 Liver abscess

Case 17 *Clostridioides (Clostridium) difficile*

Case 18 Traveller's diarrhoea

Case 19 Norovirus outbreak

Case 20 Hepatitis E

Case 21 Hepatitis C

Case 22 Pyelonephritis

Case 23 Continuous ambulatory peritoneal dialysis (CAPD) peritonitis

Case 24 BK- (polyomaviruses) induced nephropathy

Case 25 Schistosomiasis

Case 26 Meningitis

Case 27 Encephalitis

Case 28 Cerebral abscess

Case 29 Neurosurgical infection

Case 30 Progressive multifocal leukoencephalopathy (PML)

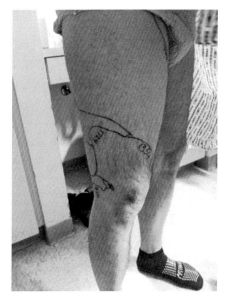

Figure 1.1 Area of rapidly spreading erythema.
Reproduced from *Infections in the Immunosuppressed Patient: An Illustrated Case-Based Approach* edited by Chandrasekhar, HP (2016). © Oxford University Press. Reproduced with permission of the Licensor through PLSclear.

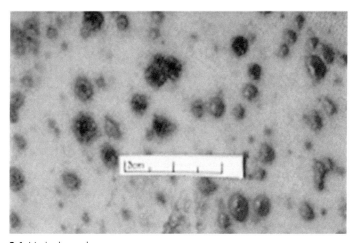

Figure 3.1 Vesicular rash.
Reproduced courtesy of David Warrell, Emeritus Professor of Tropical Medicine, Nuffield Department of Clinical Medicine, Oxford, UK.

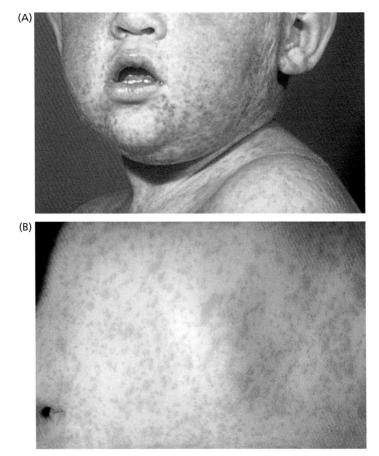

Figure 4.1 Classical rash of measles.
(A) Reproduced from CDC. ID#: 1150. 1963. https://phil.cdc.gov/details.aspx?pid=1150; (B) Reproduced from CDC/Heinz F. Eichenwald, MD. ID#3168. 1958. https://phil.cdc.gov/details.aspx?pid=3168.

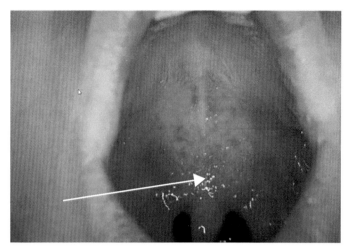

Figure 4.2 Koplik's spots on the buccal mucosa are highly suggestive of measles.
Reproduced from CDC/ Heinz F. Eichenwald, MD, 1958, https://phil.cdc.gov/Details.aspx?pid=3187.

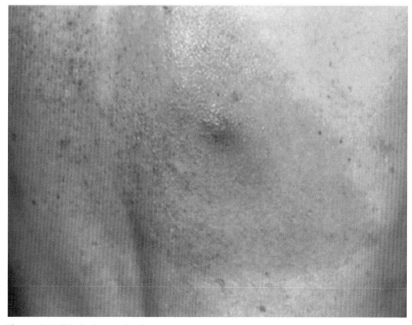

Figure 5.1 Skin lesion on back.
Reproduced with permission from Wormser GP, et al. (2010) Lyme borreliosis. In Warell DA, et al. (eds) *Oxford Textbook of Medicine, Fifth Edition.* Oxford: Oxford University Press.

How Infected Backyard Poultry Could Spread Bird Flu to People
Human Infections with Bird Flu Viruses Rare But Possible

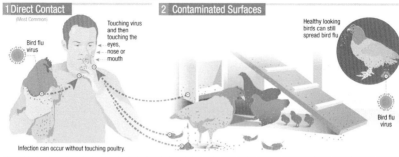

1 Direct Contact (Most Common)

Bird flu virus

Touching virus and then touching the eyes, nose or mouth

Infection can occur without touching poultry.

2 Contaminated Surfaces

Healthy looking birds can still spread bird flu

Bird flu virus

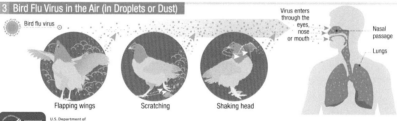

3 Bird Flu Virus in the Air (in Droplets or Dust)

Bird flu virus

Virus enters through the eyes, nose or mouth

Nasal passage

Lungs

Flapping wings   Scratching   Shaking head

U.S. Department of Health and Human Services
Centers for Disease Control and Prevention

www.cdc.gov/flu/avianflu/avian-in-humans.htm

Bird flu infections in people are rare, but possible. Most reported bird flu infections in people have happened after unprotected contact with infected birds or contaminated surfaces. This fact sheet has information about bird flu and bird flu infections in people.

Bird Flu in Birds

Wild water birds (like ducks and geese) can be infected with bird flu viruses, but usually do not get sick. Infected birds have virus in their saliva, mucous and droppings (feces). Bird flu viruses spread easily between birds. Some of these viruses can cause serious illness and death in domestic poultry (like chickens, ducks and turkeys).

Bird Flu & People

It is rare for people to get infected with bird flu viruses, but it can happen. Bird flu viruses can infect people when enough virus gets into a person's eyes, nose or mouth, or is inhaled. This might happen when virus is in the air (in droplets or possibly dust) and a person breathes it in, or when a person touches something that has virus on it and then touches their mouth, eyes or nose. (See picture on reverse side.) Most bird flu infections in people have happened after unprotected contact with infected birds or contaminated surfaces. In some cases, however, no direct contact has been reported. No human bird flu infections have been reported from proper handling of poultry meat or from eating properly cooked poultry or poultry products.

Bird flu illness in people has ranged from mild to severe. Signs and symptoms of bird flu infections in people can include: fever (temperature of 100°F [37.8°C] or greater) or feeling feverish, cough, sore throat, runny or stuffy nose, muscle or body aches, fatigue, headaches, eye redness (or conjunctivitis), and difficulty breathing. Other possible symptoms are diarrhea, nausea, and vomiting. As with seasonal flu, some people are at high risk of getting very sick from bird flu infections, including pregnant women, people with weakened immune systems and people 65 and older. Human infections with bird flu viruses usually can be treated with the same prescription drugs that are used to treat human seasonal flu viruses. These are called "flu antiviral drugs."

Bird Flu Outbreaks in Birds

Outbreaks of bird flu happen among birds from time to time. When deadly bird flu outbreaks happen in U.S. poultry, the United States Department of Agriculture (USDA) works with industry, state and other government partners to stop the outbreak so that it does not spread to other poultry. The Centers for Disease Control and Prevention works with partners to protect the public's health during these outbreaks. The risk to the public from bird flu outbreaks is low; however, because other bird flu viruses have infected people, it is possible that human infections with these viruses could occur. Risk depends on exposure. People with no contact with infected poultry or contaminated surfaces are thought to be at very low to no risk of infection. People with close or prolonged unprotected contact with infected birds or contaminated environments are thought to be at greater (though probably still low) risk of infection.

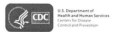

U.S. Department of Health and Human Services
Centers for Disease Control and Prevention

More information about bird flu is available at **www.cdc.gov/flu/avianflu**

Figure 8.1 Spread of avian influenza from birds to humans.
Reproduced from Center for Disease Control and Prevention (CDC). *Avian Influenza A Virus Infections in Human.* https://www.cdc.gov/flu/avianflu/avian-in-humans.htm.

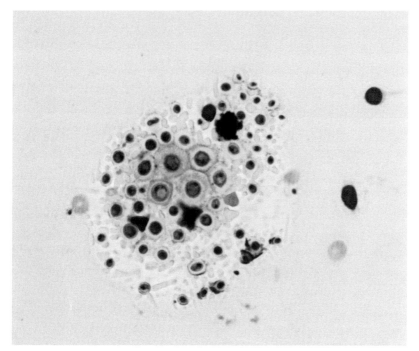

Figure 14.1 May–Grunwald stain of a cytospin preparation of a CSF sample showing yeasts subsequently identified as *C. neoformans*.
Reproduced courtesy of Michael Farrell, Beaumont Hospital, Dublin, Ireland.

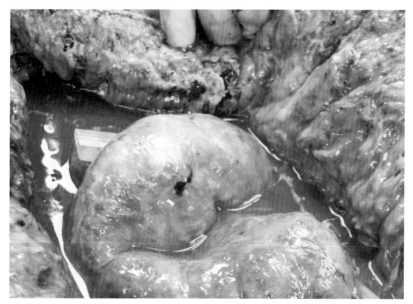

Figure 15.1 Generalized peritonitis at laparotomy with pus adherent to the colon and peritoneum.
Reproduced courtesy of Emma Tong, Royal College Surgeons in Ireland (RCSI), Ireland.

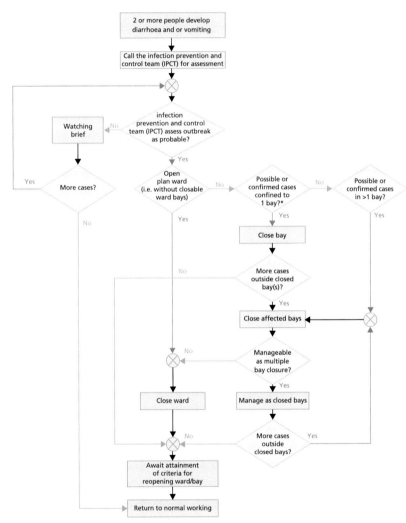

Figure 19.1 Algorithm for closure of bays or other clinical areas.

Reproduced with permission from Health Protection Scotland. (2013). *HPS Norovirus Outbreak Guidance: Preparedness, Control Measures, and Practical Considerations for Optimal Patient Safety and Service Continuation in Hospitals.* © Copyright Health Protection Scotland for the NHS National Services Scotland, the NHS Scotland and its agents.

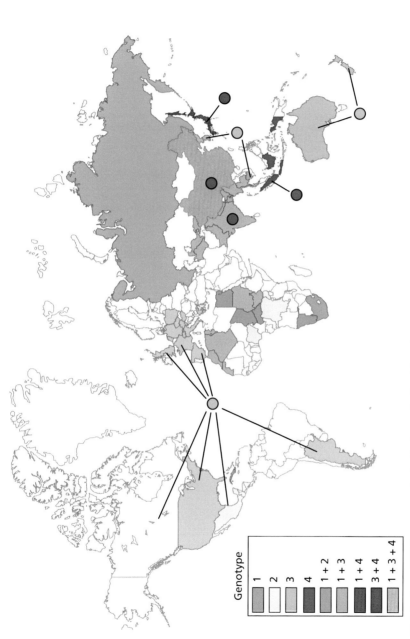

Figure 20.1 Distribution of HEV genotypes in viral isolates obtained from humans and animals (predominantly pigs). The colours used for a country and the circle associated with it represent the predominant HEV genotypes of human and animal isolates, respectively, from that country.

Reproduced with permission from Aggarwal R and Jameel S (2011). Hepatitis E. *Hepatology.* 54(6):2218–2226. DOI: 10.1002/hep.24674. Source: data from Okamoto, H. Genetic variability and evolution of hepatitis E virus. *Virus Res.* 127(2):216–28.

Genotype

1
2
3
4
1 + 2
1 + 3
1 + 4
3 + 4
1 + 3 + 4

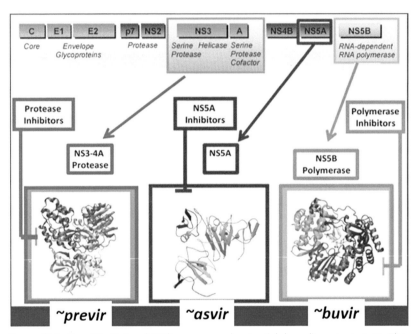

Figure 21.1 Hepatitis C virus (HCV) genome and potential drug discovery targets. The HCV RNA genome serves as a template for viral replication and as a viral messenger RNA for viral production. It is translated into a polyprotein that is cleaved by proteases. All the HCV enzymes—NS2- 3 and NS3-4A proteases, NS3 helicase, and NS5B RdRp—are essential for HCV replication, and are therefore potential drug discovery targets.

Adapted with permission from Asselah T and Marcellin P (2012). Direct acting antivirals for the treatment of chronic hepatitis C: one pill a day for tomorrow. *Liver Int*. 32 (Suppl 1):88–102. DOI: https://doi.org/10.1111/j.1478-3231.2011.02699.x.

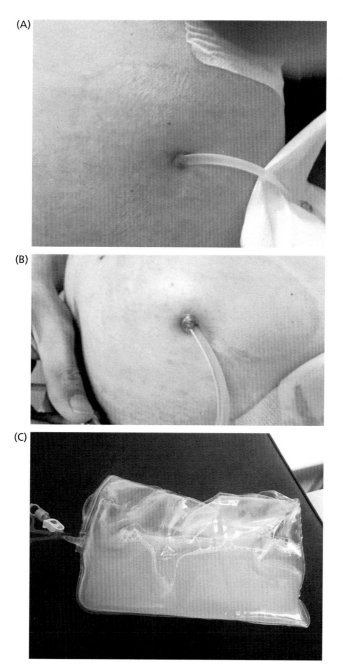

Figure 23.1 CAPD catheter exit site and peritonitis. (A). normal exit site, (B). infected exit site, (C). cloudy bag.
Reproduced courtesy of Annette Butler, Beaumont Hospital, Dublin, Ireland.

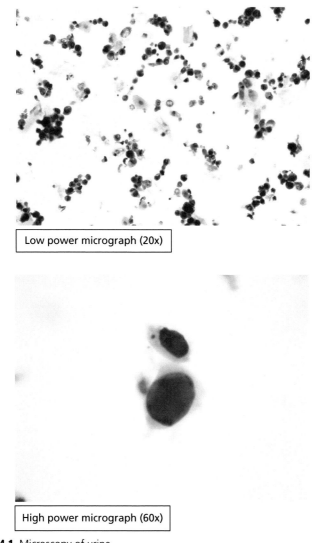

Low power micrograph (20x)

High power micrograph (60x)

Figure 24.1 Microscopy of urine.
Reproduced courtesy of Ian Roberts, Cellular Pathology, Oxford University Hospitals NHS Foundation Trust, Oxford, UK.

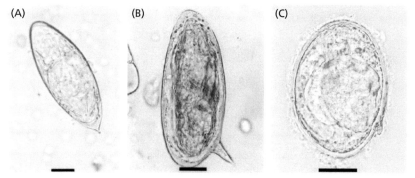

Figure 25.1 Schistosomiasis eggs. (A) *S. haematobium* (in urine); (B) *S. mansoni* (in stool); (C) *S. japonicum* (in stool). [Scale: bar = 25 μ m].
Reproduced with permission from World Health Organization. (1994). *Bench Aids for the Diagnosis of Faecal Parasites*. Geneva: World Health Organization.

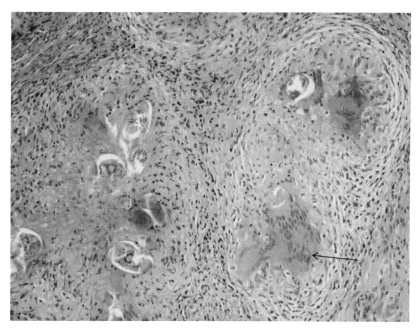

Figure 25.2 Multiple schistosoma ova associated with a granulomatous inflammatory response, including multinucleated giant cells (arrow). H&E, ×200.
Reproduced courtesy of University Hospitals Birmingham NHS Foundation Trust, UK.

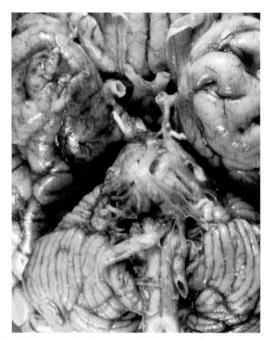

Figure 27.2 Bilateral haemorrhagic temporal lobe necrosis on post-mortem of a patient that died of HSV encephalitis.
Reproduced courtesy of Michael Farrell, Neuropathologist, Beaumont Hospital, Dublin, Ireland.

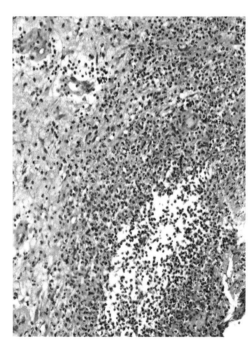

Figure 28.2 Chronic abscess with fibrous wall. Grocott staining for fungi was negative.
Reproduced courtesy of Michael Farrell, Neuropathologist, Beaumont Hospital, Dublin, Ireland.

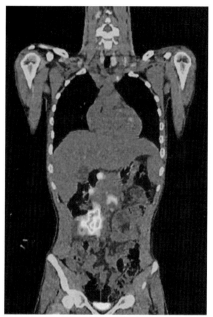
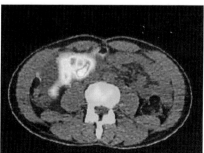

Figure 31.1 Images from PET-CT showing high uptake of ^{18}F-FDG in upper abdominal lymph nodes in a patient with fever of 8 weeks duration. No other lymphadenopathy was evident. Tuberculosis was diagnosed by histology and culture after biopsy samples obtained.

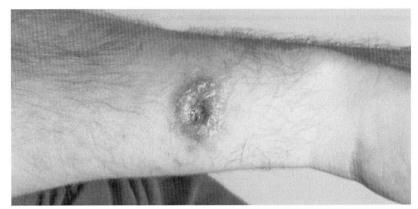

Figure 37.1 Ulcerated forearm lesion.

Reproduced courtesy of Lt Col (Prof) Mark Bailey, Consultant Physician and Professor in Infectious Diseases and Tropical Medicine, Birmingham Heartlands Hospital, Warwick Medical School, and Royal Centre for Defence Medicine, UK.

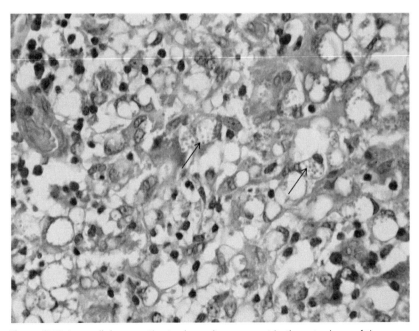

Figure 37.2 Intracellular amastigotes (arrow) are present in the cytoplasm of the histiocytes. H&E ×600.

Reproduced courtesy of University Hospitals Birmingham NHS Foundation Trust, UK.

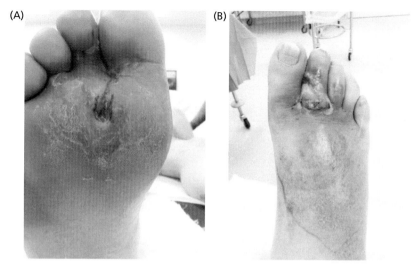

Figure 42.1 Photos of foot. (A) Plantar surface; (B) Dorsum of foot.
Reproduced courtesy of Department of Microbiology and Infectious Diseases, John Radcliffe Hospital, Oxford, UK.

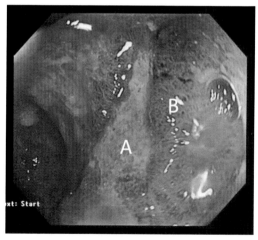

Figure 46.1 Colonoscopy showing features of CMV colitis. A mucosal ulcer (A) is surrounded by erythema (B).
Reproduced courtesy of University Hospitals Birmingham NHS Foundation Trust, UK.

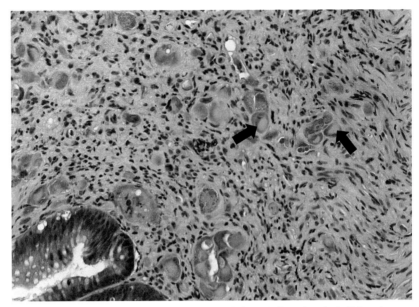

Figure 46.2 Cytomegalovirus colitis with multiple large infected endothelial and stromal cells in the lamina propria showing typical intranuclear inclusions (arrows). (HE; ×200).
Reproduced courtesy of University Hospitals Birmingham NHS Foundation Trust, UK.

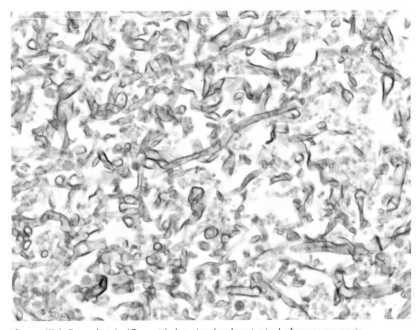

Figure 47.1 Fungal stain (Grocott) showing hyphae typical of mucormycosis.
Reproduced courtesy of Michael Farrell, Neuropathologist, Beaumont Hospital, Dublin, Ireland.

Index

Tables, figures, and boxes are indicated by an italic *t*, *f*, and *b* following the page number.

For the benefit of digital users, indexed terms that span two pages (e.g., 52–53) may, on occasion, appear on only one of those pages.